Laura Henderson
656-8303

103 Morton Rd
Oregon City OR
97045

D0747170

The All-New Pocket Encyclopedia of Calories and Nutrition

Arnold E. Bender

Revised Edition

A Fireside Book
Published by Simon & Schuster, Inc.
New York

METRIC EQUIVALENTS AND ABBREVIATIONS

Metric equivalents are approximate throughout (for example, 1oz = 28.4g; this has been rounded up to 30g throughout)

Approximate metric equivalents

1oz = 30g (= 1fl.oz)	6oz = 170g
2oz = 60g	7oz = 200g
4oz = 110g	8oz = 230g
5oz = 140g	1lb = 450g

1 liter = $1\frac{3}{4}$ pints
1 pint (20fl.oz) = 600ml (6dl)
$\frac{1}{4}$ pint (5fl.oz) = 140ml ($1\frac{1}{2}$dl)

N.B. μg = micrograms
mg = milligrams
1,000 calories = kilocalorie (kcal) or Calorie
1,000 joules = kilojoule (kJ)
1,000,000 joules = megajoule (MJ)
1 calorie = 4.2 joules

Designed and edited by
Mitchell Beazley International Limited,
Artists House, 14–15 Manette Street, London W1V 5LB

A Fireside Book published by Simon & Schuster, Inc.
Simon & Schuster Building, Rockefeller Center
1230 Avenue of the Americas, New York, New York 10020

FIRESIDE and colophon are registered trademarks of Simon & Schuster, Inc.

Photoset by MS Filmsetting Limited, Frome, Somerset, England
Printed and bound in Hong Kong by Mandarin Offset International Ltd.

1 2 3 4 5 6 7 8 9 10

Editor   David Townsend Jones
Art Editor   Ruth Levy
Production   Androulla Pavlou

Bender, Arnold E. (Arnold Eric)
    The all-new pocket encyclopedia of calories and nutrition

    Rev. ed. of: Pocket encyclopedia of calories and nutrition. 1979.
    1. Nutrition. 2. Diet. 3. Reducing diets.
4. Food—Composition—Tables. 5. Food—Caloric
content—Tables. I. Bender, Arnold E. (Arnold Eric).
Pocket encyclopedia of calories and nutrition.
II. Title. [DNLM: 1.—popular works.
2. Nutritional Requirements—popular works.
3. Nutritive Value—tables. QU 145 B458a]
RA784.B37 1985   641'.042   85-1527
ISBN 0-671-60033-8

Contents

4 List of tables

5 Foreword

6 Good food—good health
6 What is a good diet?
6 How the body utilizes food

8 The essential nutrients
8 Proteins
9 Carbohydrates
9 Fats
9 Vitamins
14 Mineral salts

16 Measuring energy: calories and joules
16 How much fuel do we need?

20 What should we eat?
20 How much of each nutrient?
20 What is RDA?
21 Which foods supply the nutrients?
33 Dietary fiber
35 Are we properly fed?
37 A sensible approach
37 Dietary goals
39 What about cholesterol?

40 Alcohol

43 Fresh or processed food?
43 Better or worse?
44 Some myths

47 Health foods and special diets
47 "Natural" foods
47 Chemical additives
48 Homemade foods
48 "Whole foods"
49 Organically grown food
50 Vitamin supplements
50 "Magic foods"
51 Pills and potions

51 Vegetarianism
52 Veganism
52 Macrobiotic diet

53 Obesity and dieting
53 Causes of obesity
54 How fat is too fat?
55 Losing weight
60 How much food?
61 What is brown fat?
61 Does dietary fiber help?
61 Children and weight

62 Questions and answers
62 General health
63 Nutrition
65 Dieting

67 Recipes for better health
67 Hors d'oeuvre
69 Soups
70 Egg and cheese dishes
74 Meat, poultry and fish dishes
78 Salads
80 Basic sauces
81 Desserts and cakes

85 Food composition and Calorie tables
85 How to use the tables
86 Dairy produce
88 Meat, poultry and game
91 Seafood
94 Vegetables
99 Fruit, nuts and seeds
103 Grain products
105 Miscellaneous
106 Homemade desserts
108 Homemade main dishes, side dishes and accompaniments
114 Nonalcoholic beverages
116 Alcoholic beverages
118 Brand names

127 Notes

List of tables

1 Nutritionally important vitamins *10*
2 Energy expenditure in Calories per minute for a 154-lb (70-kg) adult *17*
3 Daily energy balance sheets for an office worker and a manual worker—weight 145lb (66kg), height 5ft 6in (168cm) *18*
4 A representative day's diet *19*
5 US Food and Nutrition Board Recommended Daily Dietary Allowances, revised 1980 *22-23*
6 Sources of protein *24*
7 Good sources of vitamin A *25*
8 Good sources of niacin *26*
9 Good sources of vitamin B_1 *27*
10 Good sources of vitamin B_2 *27*
11 Sources of vitamin C *28-31*
12 Good sources of vitamin D *32*
13 Good sources of iron *33*
14 Good sources of calcium *34*
15 Principal sources of dietary fiber *36*
16 Moderate and excessive amounts of alcohol *39*
17 Nutritional value of alcoholic drinks *40-41*
18 Nutritional value of soft drinks *40-41*
19 Desirable weights for adults *56-57*
20 Height/weight/age table for boys of school age *58-59*
21 Height/weight/age table for girls of school age *58-59*

Food composition and calorie tables—see
CONTENTS on previous page

Foreword

The science of nutrition is steadily developing, and there is a corresponding increase in the public demand for up-to-date guidance and information. Since the first edition of the *Pocket Encyclopedia of Calories and Nutrition* was written there has been a much clearer consensus among scientists on several aspects of nutrition—the need to reduce the consumption of saturated fats, sugar and salt, for instance, and the importance of increasing the consumption of foods that supply dietary fiber.

Similarly the earlier method of assessing overweight according to the size of the body frame—which always encouraged a little cheating anyway—has been replaced by a broader range of acceptable weights. Recent evidence has shown that body weights a little above average are not a health hazard, and it is now accepted that there is a perfectly natural and normal variation between individuals.

This new edition fully reflects these and other significant changes of opinion related to advances in research worldwide, and has been comprehensively revised and updated throughout.

I would like to thank Tony Nash (Dr Nash since the first edition appeared), who initially produced the FOOD COMPOSITION AND CALORIE TABLES on a computer. I would also wish to acknowledge the lasting contributions of Corine Plough and Susannah Read, the editors of the original book, much of whose work is carried forward to this revised edition.

Arnold Bender

Good food – good health

WHAT IS A GOOD DIET?
Different people eat quite different kinds of food—fish and chips, frogs' legs, corn and beans, cassava and peanuts—and all keep quite fit. So what is really meant by a good diet? It is diet that supplies all that is necessary for growth and repair of the body tissues, the energy needed for daily activities, and all the materials needed to enable the body to work properly.

HOW THE BODY UTILIZES FOOD
Foods can be divided into those for: Growth or construction; Energy or fuel; and Function. (And since some foods we eat have little nutritional value we can add a fourth category: foods for fun.)

Growth and construction
A baby born weighing about 6½lb (3kg) might after twenty years or so weigh about 130lb (60kg). This is a result of diet. Moreover, there is a continuous process of replacing worn-out tissue, even in young people. The materials needed for such construction and repair are *mineral salts* and *proteins*.

Mineral salts, especially calcium and phosphate, together with smaller amounts of other minerals such as magnesium and fluoride, are needed to construct the framework of the body, the skeleton. Calcium cannot be absorbed from the diet into the bloodstream unless vitamin D is present, and this vitamin also helps the deposition of calcium to form bones. Muscles, vital organs, skin and the blood, which carries nutrients around the body, are all made of protein, and since we cannot synthesize protein we have to eat it instead.

Energy and fuel
To explain what nutrition and body function are all about, the body can be likened to an automobile. The structure—the bodywork and engine—is made largely of protein and minerals, and fuel is needed to supply the energy to make it go. This comes mainly from *carbohydrate* and *fat*. Carbohydrate is the principal fuel for the body; this is its only function. A small proportion of fats is used in tissue structure, but by far the greater part is used for fuel. Additionally, any protein that is not needed for construction can be burned to supply energy.

If you take on board an automobile more gas than is

needed it has to be stored in cans in the trunk. If you eat more energy foods than the body needs, the excess has to be stored as fat in various parts of the body (not excluding the trunk!).

On the other hand, if you fail to take in enough fuel you will gradually use up all the reserves and empty the tank. The body has the additional property of being able to burn up some of its own structural tissues, the muscle proteins, rather as if the automobile were fitted with wooden seats that could be burned for fuel in an emergency. When all the stored fuel is used and the tanks are empty, and all the disposable tissues have been used up for fuel, then the automobile cannot go—the body cannot continue to function.

Fortunately most people have a built-in fuel-filling system: they feel hungry when fuel is needed and rarely allow the tank to empty. On the contrary, they are more likely to take too much in and the reserves may grow dangerously large.

Function

Continuing the automobile analogy, fuel and engine alone are not enough. They cannot work without spark plugs—the body cannot function without *vitamins*. These are neither materials of construction nor fuel but are needed in very small amounts to permit proper functioning of the body. Some vitamins require the joint function of mineral salts, so these may be considered both structural and functional.

Finally, the importance of *dietary fiber*, or roughage, should also be mentioned. This is a particular type of indigestible carbohydrate material without which the intestine cannot function properly.

7

The essential nutrients

PROTEINS

Proteins are found in foods as diverse as milk, peas, liver, eggs, bread, potatoes and fish. In fact, since proteins are the basis of all living tissues, everything that is grown, plant and animal, contains some protein unless the food has been extracted from its original source. For example, when olive oil is pressed from the olive or sugar extracted from the cane, what is obtained is a pure fat and a pure carbohydrate, although the original olive and the sugar cane did contain some protein. So even cabbage and rhubarb—90 percent water—contain a little protein (2-3 percent), whereas wheat, corn and rice contain about 10 percent, and meat and fish are called rich sources because they contain 20 percent protein.

To put these figures into perspective, a good diet should contain 5-10 percent protein, although most of us prefer to eat a diet of 10-12 percent protein, which is the approximate norm.

You may wonder how proteins from such diverse sources can be used to make human flesh, blood, liver and lungs. The answer is that all proteins are made of 20 basic units, the amino acids, linked together in a variety of combinations. During the process of digestion the proteins are broken down into their constituent amino acids, absorbed into the bloodstream and travel around the body to the places where they are needed. Here they are rebuilt into the particular proteins needed for kidneys, heart, glands and all the other tissues.

So any protein can be used to make human protein. Some, however, must be more useful than others. For example, would it not be more efficient if we were all cannibals so that the protein we ate was the same composition as the protein in the body? Only to a limited extent. Firstly, in the continuous process of breakdown and repair that goes on, tissues like heart and intestine are being broken down and replaced much faster than the muscles and very much faster than the skin and bones, so to eat representative samples of human tissue would not be all that practical. Secondly, it is only when we are eating the bare minimum amount of protein—about $1\frac{1}{2}$ oz (45g) a day—that we need worry whether the proportions of amino acids in the protein closely resemble those of the body. In the industrialized world we eat two or three times as much protein as this, so even if the amino acid makeup differs considerably from our requirements, quantity makes up for quality. The body simply selects those amino acids it needs from those that are eaten, and the rest are burned off to provide energy.

CARBOHYDRATES

These are the starchy foods and sugars that make up the greater part of our cereals, pastas, cakes and biscuits. In round figures our diet is about 50 percent carbohydrate, 40 percent fat and 10 percent protein. About one-third of the carbohydrate is sugar—half of this is taken in cups of tea and coffee, and the rest in manufactured and cooked foods.

Bread, the commonest food in many countries, consists of 50 percent carbohydrate, 10 percent protein and 2 percent fat, the rest being water. Bread is often called a starchy food, but from the point of view of protein we could live on bread alone.

Sugar, on the other hand, contains nothing but carbohydrate—it is, in fact, a very pure chemical substance. So when we make flour confectionery by mixing flour (at 10 percent protein) with sugar (zero protein) and fat (also zero protein) we are diluting a good food to a point where it sometimes contributes little to the diet other than energy, with only traces of minerals, vitamins and protein. These must be considered as fun foods rather than as sources of any particular nutrients.

FATS

Fats are fairly obvious as butter, margarine, salad oil and cooking fat, but also many other foods contain fat. Bread has already been mentioned as containing about 2 percent fat; fancy breads can contain more than that, and the level can go as high as 30 percent in some crackers. Then there are milk and cheese, fatty meats and fatty fish. Even in very lean meat there is as much as 10 percent fat between the muscle fibers. Consequently many foods that are not themselves fats do contain quite a lot of fat.

A small amount of fat is essential in the diet—about 10 percent, failing which certain vitamins, such as vitamins A and D, cannot be absorbed into the bloodstream from the digestive tract. In Western communities about 40 percent of the energy we consume is fat. As discussed later, this is thought to be too much for good health. Certainly fat helps the food go down—just imagine trying to swallow dry bread in any quantity—and in many foods the greater part of the flavor is in the fatty part. A further point is that fats are a more concentrated form of energy than carbohydrates and proteins, so that if a diet is very low in fat it will have to be bulkier and will often be too bulky for comfort.

VITAMINS

There are 13 vitamins of known importance to man (Table 1). All are essential to life, but eight are of special

1 Nutritionally important vitamins

Number	Name	
A	Retinol (in animal foods) Carotene (in plant foods)	
B_1	Thiamine	
B_2	Riboflavin	
—	Niacin or nicotinic acid	B-complex
—	Folic acid or Folacin	group
B_6	Pyridoxine	
C	Ascorbic acid	
D	Cholecalciferol	

Less important vitamins

E	Tocopherol
K	Menaphthone
—	Pantothenic acid
B_{12}	Cyanocobalamin
H	Biotin

nutritional importance since they are in short supply in some communities and some individuals. Deficiencies of the other vitamins are caused not so much through a dietary shortage but because the subject suffers from some disease or is unable to absorb the vitamins from the food.

The nutritionally important vitamins

Vitamin A is needed for growth and to keep the cells that line the various passages of the body in their normal moist condition. Although well-fed people have about two years' supply of the vitamin in their livers, in many developing countries, especially in the southeast Pacific and Middle East, there is a widespread shortage which results in cells becoming dry and hard. If this happens in the eye it damages the cornea and eventually leads to blindness. Another function of vitamin A is to enable us to see in dim light; when the supply is inadequate night blindness results. It is not, however, involved in vision in full light.

Vitamin A is found in animal foods as retinol, the form used in our bodies. In plant foods it exists in the form of carotene, which is converted into retinol in the walls of the intestine. It is plentiful in a wide variety of foods, including milk, butter, yellow and orange fruit, green vegetables, and particularly in liver and carrots. One carrot weighing 2oz (60g) can contain a 3-day supply of carotene.

B vitamins can be considered together since some have parallel functions and also often occur together in the same foods. For example, meat and cereals contain vitamin B_1, niacin and some vitamin B_2, and it is present in large amounts in liver and in milk.

So far as function is concerned, vitamins B_1, B_2 and niacin are involved at different stages in the release of energy from foods. The energy is not liberated suddenly, just as an automobile does not function by setting the gasoline ablaze, but through a complex 20-stage system with the aid of these three vitamins.

Vitamin B_6 is concerned with reconstituting amino acids derived from food protein into the proteins of the body. Good sources include meat, especially liver, green vegetables and unrefined cereals.

Folic acid is also found in a wide variety of foods, especially liver and many vegetables; problems seldom arise from a shortage of it. A deficiency results in anemia.

B-vitamin-deficiency diseases are various, and some of them can be fatal. A serious and prolonged shortage of vitamin B_1 results in beriberi. This disease was very common, and still exists in Far Eastern countries. Victims have difficulty in walking because of damage to the nerves, and the heart is affected. It was shown to be a nutritional disease in the Japanese Navy as long ago as 1883, caused by relying on white rice as the main part of the diet. Whole-grain (or brown) rice contains plenty of vitamin B_1, but it is removed during milling to white rice. This also happens when wheat is milled to white flour, but Western countries obtain their vitamin B_1 from so many other foods that beriberi never occurs. Eastern sufferers do not get these other foods, so beriberi is associated with rice-eating communities.

Pellagra results from a serious deficiency of niacin. It was described 250 years ago and literally means, in Italian, rough skin. This is because it looks like a specific type of dermatitis, particularly on the face, neck and arms, which are exposed to light; there is damage also to the digestive system and the brain. It was many years before the precise dietary problem was identified—at one time it was thought to be caused by harmful substances in corn because it is common in corn-eating areas, then by protein shortage, and, in the 1940s, it was thought to be caused by niacin deficiency. In fact all three theories are correct. One of the amino acids that is present in protein, namely tryptophan, is converted into niacin in the body—and corn is relatively short of both.

Vitamin B_2 and B_6 deficiency may cause cracking of the skin at the corners of the mouth, and soreness of the lips and tongue.

Vitamin C or, rather, scurvy caused by a shortage of vitamin C, has a long history. The vitamin is found in fruit and vegetables, and is largely destroyed by drying and more slowly during storage.

The people who suffered most from scurvy were sailors who, being away from land for months or even years, had little fresh food, and sometimes no fruit and vegetables at all. When Vasco da Gama in 1497 sailed around the Cape of Good Hope, 100 out of his crew of 160 died of scurvy. It became known early in the sixteenth century that the juice of certain leaves was a cure, and successful explorers such as Captain Cook stopped at every opportunity to take on board fruit and vegetables. Scurvy was eliminated in the British Navy after 1795 by providing lime juice— hence the name of "limeys" for Britishers.

Although vitamin C is present in all fruit and vegetables the amounts vary enormously, and a lot can be lost in processing and cooking. Black currants, for example, are an extremely rich source containing as much as 200mg per $3\frac{1}{2}$oz (100g), while apples contain only about 5mg per $3\frac{1}{2}$oz (100g). Oranges contain about 50mg each and leafy vegetables contain 30 to 100mg per $3\frac{1}{2}$oz (100g).

Figures given for vitamin C in foods are very approximate because it is so readily lost. First, we find that the amount originally present in the fresh food can vary a great deal depending on the variety of plant, soil, climate, fertilizer and growing conditions; the fruit on the sunny side of the tree may contain more vitamin C than the rest. Next, there is a steady loss once the crop has been harvested because of self-destruction by an enzyme present in the fruit or vegetable. In the living plant this is kept separate, but when the leaf begins to wilt after cropping or the fruit is slightly bruised, especially in mechanical harvesting and transport, the enzyme comes into contact with the vitamin and it is steadily destroyed.

The next loss takes place during cooking, when the greater part can be washed out into the water, the amount depending, of course, on how finely the food is chopped. There is 80 or 90 percent loss from chopped cabbage, but only 20 or 30 percent loss from whole potatoes. Much of this can be recovered from the water, so it is sound practice to use the water for gravies.

The final loss takes place because of oxidation by air when the food is kept hot before eating. Mashed potato, for example, can lose half its remaining vitamin C if kept hot for 20 minutes.

Despite this enormous loss, there is no great likelihood of scurvy in most countries since half an orange will provide nearly all the vitamin C needed for a day. Most people eat some vegetables, however badly they may be cooked, and fruit, and there is even a little in milk and in jam. Scurvy is the result of severe deficiency; the effects of long-term very slight shortages are unclear.

Vitamin D has the unique distinction of being a nutrient that can be synthesized in the skin under the influence of sunlight. We do not know how much is made under the skin: it obviously depends on how much sunlight reaches how much skin, so we cannot say exactly how much ought to be consumed. It is needed for both absorption of calcium from the diet into the bloodstream and for the deposition of calcium on the bones.

Therefore a deficiency in growing children, who need to form new bone, and adolescents who are undergoing a growth spurt, can cause rickets. A deficiency is also possible in adults, not from lack of new bone growth but through loss of calcium from existing bones. In adults it is termed osteomalacia and is found in women on a poor diet, sheltered from sunlight by living largely indoors and with repeated pregnancies that call for extra calcium for the growing infant. Such deficiencies in pregnant women are rare in the industrialized world but are common in some developing countries. Probably the greater problem in industrialized countries is that of elderly housebound people, who are consequently without the benefit of sunshine and who, at the same time, eat a diet restricted in variety and particularly lacking in ready-made vitamin D. Problems also occur in the UK in some young children because of lack of the vitamin in their diet, and also, for reasons not yet understood, among adolescent Asian children.

Not many foods contain vitamin D. Fatty fish are a good source, there is some in eggs and butter, and it is added to margarine and milk.

Vitamin B₆ (pyridoxine) in large doses may help to alleviate premenstrual syndrome (PMS). The RDA (see page 20) is only about 2 mg (using the US RDA figure), while the dose used for PMS is 50-100 mg a day for several months. Such large doses cannot simply be correcting a vitamin deficiency but must be functioning, if at all, like a medical drug. The value of B_6 in PMS is therefore by no means certain and it is still under trial.

Folacin is particularly necessary during pregnancy to supply the rapidly growing fetus, and is prescribed by some doctors. There is considerable research into the possibility that a shortage of folic acid in the very first few weeks of pregnancy may be the cause of spina bifida (neural tube defect) in newborn babies. The problem here is that the effects of a shortage occur so early in pregnancy that the vitamin is needed *before* pregnancy occurs.

The less important vitamins

Many people around the world suffer deficiencies of the vitamins discussed above, while deficiencies of the other vitamins are very rare.

For example, nobody, even in the developing countries, has ever been shown to suffer from a shortage of vitamin E. A deficiency can be created in the laboratory on controlled diets, or can occur after surgery or in diseases that prevent absorption of the vitamin, but it seems that all diets, however poor, contain enough.

Another vitamin that almost never seems to be in short supply is vitamin H, or biotin. We do know that it can become linked to raw egg white and pass straight through the intestine without being absorbed, but it seems you would have to eat an extraordinary diet to create a deficiency, as illustrated by the first and almost only case, which was reported from the United States in 1943. This was an egg farmer who ate six dozen raw eggs a week washed down with a daily dose of 4 quarts (4.5 litres) of red wine (his wife and children left him). He developed a type of dermatitis and finished up in the hospital. Since there are many types of dermatitis he was treated with one substance after another until finally he responded to vitamin H. Such eccentrics often provide as much scientific data as carefully planned laboratory experiments.

A dietary shortage of vitamin B_{12} is also very rare; however, some people are unable to absorb it and this is the cause of pernicious anemia.

MINERAL SALTS

A very large number of mineral salts is needed, but only a few are likely to be undersupplied: these are iron, calcium, iodine, fluorine and zinc.

The nutritionally important minerals

Iron is part of the red coloring material of the blood and when it is in short supply iron-deficiency anemia results. Mild anemia is very common, particularly among women, since the loss of blood in menstruation means a loss of iron from the body. It is so common that anemia is often regarded as the main nutritional deficiency in well-fed countries, but there are recent medical suggestions that mild anemia is not a problem but just a normal variation between people. It is only when the blood hemoglobin falls well below normal levels that the anemia becomes severe enough to be regarded as ill health.

Unfortunately iron is not well absorbed from foods: often only 10 percent or less is absorbed. Meat and animal products such as liver and other organ meats are particularly rich in iron that is reasonably well absorbed. Some other foods, such as curry powder, black molasses and cocoa, are relatively rich in iron, but the amount absorbed is very variable and is certainly far less than that absorbed from meat. Vitamin C in amounts of 50-100mg greatly assists the absorption of iron from foods eaten at the same meal.

Calcium itself is usually adequately supplied—the problem is ensuring sufficient vitamin D to help absorb it. We need to consume about one gram of calcium a day, and milk and cheese are the only foods particularly rich in this mineral, unless bread is fortified as in some countries.

Iodine is not obtained in sufficient quantity in certain areas and this shortage results in goiter: the thyroid gland, located in the throat, enlarges and can become big enough to be seen as a large swelling. The iodine content of plant and animal foods depends on how much there is in the soil, and there is not much in limestone areas, so that goiter is a local problem; it was called "Derbyshire neck" when it was common in that part of England.

The only rich source of iodine in the diet is fish.

Fluorine is a mineral salt, the importance of which lies in protecting teeth from decay. It is always present in bones, teeth and skin, and therefore is a dietary essential like many other minerals. It has been shown in many parts of the world that where the drinking water has about one part of fluorine per million parts of water dental decay is much less than in areas where there are only traces. That is why it is added to water in some places.

Zinc provides an example of how recent research has revealed properties of nutrients not previously suspected. It was as late as 1960 that zinc deficiency was shown to be a problem in some parts of the world. A deficiency has adverse effects on fertility and delays sexual development in young men. There are traces of zinc in most foods, and good sources include meat and meat by-products, and shellfish.

The less important minerals

Other minerals are rarely, if ever, in short supply: for example, phosphate, sulphate, chloride, sodium, potassium and magnesium are all needed but are plentiful in almost every diet. Although phosphate has often been used as a general "tonic," there is never any likelihood of a shortage and, in fact, food regulations in some countries prevent manufacturers making any claims for its presence in their products. It is added as a processing aid to meat products such as poultry and sausages because it holds water and keeps them juicy and soft. Magnesium is found in small but adequate amounts in many foods; bran, cocoa and some nuts are rich sources.

It is true of all the nutrients that we are unsure of the effects of long-term very slight deficiencies. Mild shortages may give rise to vague symptoms that are more than difficult to diagnose.

So how can we make sure that we are getting an adequate amount of all the nutrients described above, and what quantity of which foods will supply it? These questions, together with guidelines for a sensible diet, will be dealt with in WHAT SHOULD WE EAT, pages 20–39.

15

Measuring energy: calories and joules

The energy taken in as food and the energy spent in living are measured in calories and, nowadays, in joules. Both the calorie and joule are rather small units to work with, so we use a unit of 1,000 calories called a kilocalorie (kcal), or Calorie with a capital "C"; a unit of 1,000 joules called a kilojoule (kJ); and a unit of a million joules called a megajoule (MJ). In practice, "calorie" is often written when strictly it should be "Calorie."

One calorie is approximately 4 joules (to be precise, 4.2), so multiplying Calories (kilocalories) by four gives kilojoules.

The energy of food is converted into work with only about 25 percent efficiency; the rest is wasted as heat. Although this may seem rather inefficient, it is about as efficient as the internal combustion engine and much better than the steam engine.

HOW MUCH FUEL DO WE NEED?

The average adult eats and spends about 2,500 Calories (10,000 kilojoules) per day. The energy content of 1g of starch or sugar or any other carbohydrate is 4 Calories (16 kilojoules); that of 1g of protein is 4 Calories (17 kilojoules). (The difference between 16 and 17 is because of rounding off.) The energy content of 1g of fat or oil is 9 Calories (37 kilojoules). That is why fats are a more concentrated form of fuel and why one would need to eat a much bulkier diet to get the same energy from a carbohydrate diet. A loaf of bread weighing just over 1lb (480g) contains, in round figures, 250g starch, 50g protein and 10g fat (plus iron, calcium, and B vitamins). This would supply 1,000 Calories (4,000 kilojoules) from carbohydrate, 200 Calories (850 kilojoules) from protein and 90 Calories (375 kilojoules) from fat—a total of 1,290 Calories (5.25 megajoules) or about half the average daily need of energy.

Table 2 lists a variety of daily, recreational and maximum-effort activities, and shows the energy expenditure per minute of a 154-lb (70-kg) adult on each. Needless to say, cycling and playing games require more energy than walking slowly. If you want to burn up a lot of energy you don't have to ski uphill or walk in loose snow: try running upstairs, which will use up about 20 Calories (80 kilojoules) per minute.

Table 3 is a daily balance sheet of energy input and expenditure for an office worker and for someone employed in heavy manual work. The table gives Calorie expenditure per minute for each of the office worker's activities and also the total time spent in each activity, so that total daily energy output may be arrived at. As the table shows, even at complete rest he spends 1.1 Calories (4.4 kilojoules) per minute keeping body and soul together, and standing puts up the cost to about 2 Calories

2 Energy expenditure in Calories per minute for a 154-lb (70-kg) adult

Daily activities	Calories per minute
Washing and dressing	2.6–3.0
Walking slowly	2.9
Walking quickly	5.2
Sitting	1.5
Sitting and writing	2.0
Driving automobile	2.8
Driving motorcycle	3.4
Sweeping floor	1.7
Ironing	4.2
Polishing floor	4.8
Recreation	
Cycling slowly	4.5
Cycling quickly	11.1
Digging	8.6
Playing tennis	7.1
Playing soccer	8.9
Baseball (fielding)	3.9
Baseball (pitching)	5.2
Baseball (striking)	6.0
Maximum efforts	
Planing hardwood	9
Shoveling earth	10
Sculling at 315ft (97m)/min	11
Swimming at 179ft (55m)/min	14
Climbing with load	13
Skiing uphill	19
Walking in loose snow	20

3 Daily energy balance sheet of an office worker
Weight 145 lb (66 kg), height 5 ft 6 in (168 cm)

	Time	Cal/min	Cal*	MJ
Sleep	8 hrs	1.1	530	2.2
Off work				
Light sedentary activity	4 hrs	1.48	360	1.5
Washing and dressing	½ hr	3.0	90	0.4
Light domestic work	1 hr	3.0	180	0.8
Walking	1 hr	6.6	400	1.7
Gardening	25 mins	4.8	120	0.5
Standing	20 mins	1.56	30	0.1
At work				
Sitting activities	3 hrs 10 mins	1.65	320	1.3
Standing activities	3 hrs 40 mins	1.9	420	1.8
Walking	12 mins	6.6	80	0.3
TOTALS				
Sleeping			530	2.2
Total working			820	3.4
Total off work			1180	4.9
Total			**2530**	**10.6**
Basal metabolic rate			1680	7.0
Energy intake calculated from diet			2620	11.0

Daily energy balance sheet of a manual worker
Weight 145 lb (66 kg), height 5 ft 6 in (168 cm)

	Cal	MJ
Sleeping	530	2.2
Work	1700	7.1
Remainder	1560	6.5
Total	**3790**	**15.8**
Basal metabolic rate	1680	7.0
Energy intake calculated from diet	3990	16.7

Total Calories per day (mean of 7 days' measurements)

4 A representative day's diet

Food	Quantity	Energy		Protein
		Cal	MJ	g
Milk	14fl.oz (420ml)	350	1.5	18
Cheese	½oz (15g)	60	0.2	4
Bread & cereals	9oz (270g)	740	3.0	19
Meats	6oz (170g)	420	1.8	21
Fats	1½oz (45g)	370	1.5	0
Sugar & preserves	2½oz (75g)	280	1.2	0
Vegetables	12oz (340g)	180	0.8	7
Fruit	5oz (140g)	60	0.3	1
Totals		**2400**	**10.1**	**66**

(8 kilojoules). (Of course, all the figures given are only averages; some people are more efficient and more economical in their movements, while others are awkward and waste a lot of effort.)

The foods shown in Table 4 would be a representative day's meals, providing about 70g protein and 2,500 Calories (10.5 megajoules).

If your body weight is not changing then you must be taking in the same amount of fuel in the form of food as you are spending in activity (resting metabolism, daily work and recreation). If you are gaining weight you must be taking in more than you are spending; if you take in less you will lose weight. Later on the problems of obesity and dieting are discussed in OBESITY AND DIETING (pages 53-61), but it is a fact of life that anyone gaining weight is eating more than he or she is using.

What should
we eat?

HOW MUCH OF EACH NUTRIENT?

We eat food, not nutrients, but we need to know how much of each nutrient we require so that we can find how much of which foods we should eat. It is possible to get a good diet—which means to obtain all the essential nutrients—from diets as different as those based on meat and two vegetables, rice and fish, or caterpillars and corn (adequately supplemented with smaller amounts of other foods), since we can get the nutrients we need from very different sources. There is no such thing as a perfect diet, but there are very many good diets adapted to individual likes and dislikes.

It is very difficult, and in the present state of knowledge impossible, to find out exactly what each individual needs—we differ so much from one another. The best that we can do, by examining diets eaten by people who appear to be perfectly well and by experimenting on a limited number of people, is to arrive at figures for the *average* nutritional requirements. It is then possible by adding a safety margin to arrive at an amount that will be enough for everyone—those with low, average and above average needs. If we eat a little of everything, all our needs for the various nutrients are most likely to be met.

WHAT IS RDA?

RDA stands for Recommended Daily Allowances. They are the amounts of each nutrient that would satisfy the daily needs of everyone, including those whose needs are above average. They are calculated by measuring in the laboratory the needs of volunteers and taking an average, then adding an extra 20 percent, which is enough for everyone.

RDA's apply only to population groups. They do *not* apply to individuals; an individual person might need 20 percent less than average, which is 40 percent less than the RDA.

They are used for planning and procuring food supplies for population groups, interpreting food-composition records, establishing standards for public assistance programs, developing nutrition education programs, and establishing guidelines for nutritional labeling of foods.

Nutrient requirements, and therefore recommended intakes, differ with sex, age, weight and activity. The extra 20 percent that is added to the average measured requirements does not apply to energy—otherwise people would presumably get fatter—but to vitamins, minerals and proteins. In any case, people vary enormously in their individual energy expenditure and therefore in their energy needs, and unless they are gaining or losing weight, appetite acts as a mechanism to ensure that their energy intake satisfies their needs.

Although RDA's are calculated on a daily basis, there is no need to worry about getting our nutrients every single day, because our bodies carry a reasonably good reserve of everything we need nutritionally. But there is neither any harm nor, indeed, any benefit to be gained in taking more than the RDA of nutrients.

In fact, those with average needs would get more than their requirements if their diet simply supplied the RDA; even a single carrot, for example, will supply far more than the RDA of vitamin A. However, while there is no harm in consuming more nutrients than we need from food, it is possible to consume excessive and possibly harmful amounts from an overdosage of vitamin preparations.

Measurements of human requirements for nutrients are difficult and complicated. They are made on a sample of only a few people, so the figures cannot be totally accurate. They depend to some extent on the opinions of the particular committee concerned, and there are some variations between tables published in different countries.

In the USA, the Committee on Dietary Allowances is appointed by the Food and Nutrition Board of the National Research Council usually on a 4-year cycle so as to take advantage of new information in periodically updating the figures. This procedure can mean that a new committee may hold different opinions from its predecessor, which accounts for some of the differences between tables published at different times.

The first edition was published in 1943 and gave as its objective: "...providing standards to serve as a goal for good nutrition." The most recent table (1980) is printed on pages 22-23 (Table 5). For the purposes of nutritional labeling, RDA's for some of the groups are averaged, and the table is titled *United States Recommended Daily Allowances (USRDA)*. Nutrients in foods are expressed as a percentage of these figures.

WHICH FOODS SUPPLY THE NUTRIENTS?
A look around the supermarket shelves shows what an enormous number of foods are available to us. Except for sugar and starch, which are carbohydrates only, and fats, most foods supply several nutrients. Some foods, however, are richer sources of protein or vitamins or minerals than others.

Energy
Energy is never a problem: almost everyone eats enough to satisfy their appetite and thus satisfy their needs for

5 United States Food and Nutrition Board Recommended Daily Dietary Allowances, revised 1980

Age	Infants 0.0-0.5	0.5-1.0	1-3	Children 4-6	7-10	Males 11-14	15-18
Weight (lb)	13	20	29	44	62	99	145
Weight (kg)	6	9	13	20	28	45	66
Height (in)	24	28	35	44	52	62	69
Height (cm)	60	71	90	112	132	157	176
Protein (g)	kg × 2.2	kg × 2.0	23	30	34	45	56
Vitamins							
▲ Vit. A (μg RE)	420	400	400	500	700	1000	1000
Vit. D (μg)	10	10	10	10	10	10	10
● Vit. E (mg TE)	3	4	5	6	7	8	10
Vit. C (mg)	35	35	45	45	45	50	60
Thiamine (mg)	0.3	0.5	0.7	0.9	1.2	1.4	1.4
Riboflavin (mg)	0.4	0.6	0.8	1.0	1.4	1.6	1.7
■ Niacin (mg NE)	6	8	9	11	16	18	18
Vit. B₆ (mg)	0.3	0.6	0.9	1.3	1.6	1.8	2.0
Folacin (μg)	30	45	100	200	300	400	400
Vitamin B₁₂ (μg)	0.5	1.5	2.0	2.5	3.0	3.0	3.0
Minerals							
Calcium (mg)	360	540	800	800	800	1200	1200
Phosphorus (mg)	240	360	800	800	800	1200	1200
Magnesium (mg)	50	70	150	200	250	350	400
Iron (mg)	10	15	15	10	10	18	18
Zinc (mg)	3	5	10	10	10	15	15
Iodine (μg)	40	50	70	90	120	150	150

▲ RE = retinol equivalent
● TE = tocopherol equivalent
■ NE = niacin equivalent

energy. On the contrary, the problem is that some people eat too much.

Protein

Nor does protein present a problem, because if we eat enough food to satisfy our energy needs we will automati-

| Males (contd) | | | Females | | | | | Preg-nant | Lac-tating |
19-22	23-50	51+	11-14	15-18	19-22	23-50	51+		
154	154	154	101	120	120	120	120		
70	70	70	46	55	55	55	55		
70	70	70	62	64	64	64	64		
178	178	178	157	163	163	163	163		
56	56	56	46	46	44	44	44	+ 30	+ 20
1000	1000	1000	800	800	800	800	800	+ 200	+ 400
7.5	5	5	10	10	7.5	5	5	+ 5	+ 5
10	10	10	8	8	8	8	8	+ 2	+ 3
60	60	60	50	60	60	60	60	+ 20	+ 40
1.5	1.4	1.2	1.1	1.1	1.1	1.0	1.0	+ 0.4	+ 0.5
1.7	1.6	1.4	1.3	1.3	1.3	1.2	1.2	+ 0.3	+ 0.5
19	18	16	15	14	14	13	13	+ 2	+ 5
2.2	2.2	2.2	1.8	2.0	2.0	2.0	2.0	+ 0.6	+ 0.5
400	400	400	400	400	400	400	400	+ 400	+ 100
3.0	3.0	3.0	3.0	3.0	3.0	3.0	3.0	+ 1.0	+ 1.0
800	800	800	1200	1200	800	800	800	+ 400	+ 400
800	800	800	1200	1200	800	800	800	+ 400	+ 400
350	350	350	300	300	300	300	300	+ 150	+ 150
10	10	10	18	18	18	18	10	high	high
15	15	15	15	15	15	15	15	+ 5	+ 10
150	150	150	150	150	150	150	150	+ 25	+ 50

Habitual American diets cannot supply sufficient iron for pregnant women, and 30-60mg of supplemental iron is recommended. Continued supplementation for 2-3 months after the birth is advisable in order to replenish stores depleted by pregnancy.

cally get enough protein. The only way we could go short of protein is if we took a substantial part of our energy as empty calories—that is, from foods which have little or no nutritional value: too much sugar, too much fat and too much alcohol. (For more about alcohol see the section on ALCOHOL, pages 40-42.) With the usual amounts of sugar, fat and alcohol that are consumed by the average person we still get at least twice as much protein as we need.

Much protein comes from cereals. Bread, flour and foods made from wheat, together with rice, barley, oats and corn, all contain roughly 10 percent protein. There are especially rich sources of protein such as meat, fish, eggs, milk and cheese; even foods rather low in protein such as vegetables and potatoes contribute to the total intake.

Table 6 shows some sources of protein.

Vitamins

We cannot be so certain that our vitamin intake is adequate, although given the types of food eaten in the Western world it is most unlikely that there would be a shortage severe enough to give rise to deficiency diseases. What is more likely is that we might not get quite enough and be below maximum efficiency and optimum health without realising it. Then when some infection such as influenza comes along or we break a leg it might take longer to recover. This is more than difficult to prove and the only way to make sure that we are getting enough is to eat all the right foods.

The water-soluble vitamins of the B complex and vitamin C, unlike vitamins A and D, are not much stored in the body, so a deficiency can arise within a few weeks. While it is by no means essential to consume these vitamins every day at every meal, it is advisable to consume them fairly regularly. Vitamins A and D, on the other hand, could, if one wanted, be eaten once a week or

6 Sources of protein

Food	Protein:	g/oz*	g/100g†
Dried skim-milk		10	35
Sunflower seeds		8	28
Peanuts		8	28
Cheese (Cheddar)		7	25
Dried whole milk		7	25
Green peas (dry)		7	25
Beans (dry)		7	25
Almonds		6	21
Beef		5	18
Codfish		5	18
Evaporated milk		2	7
Green peas (fresh)		1.6	6
Milk		0.9	3

*grams of protein per oz †grams of protein per 100g

even less frequently.

Vitamin A The needs of an adult will be satisfied with about 750 micrograms of this vitamin a day. It is found in very large amounts in carrots and liver: $3\frac{1}{2}$oz (100g) of either would keep us going for a week or more. Milk, butter, egg yolk, cheese, tomatoes, all green vegetables, and yellow and orange fruit such as apricots, peaches and melons also supply vitamin A. Countries in which dairy produce and meat supplies are scarce rely heavily upon vegetable and fruit sources as an alternative. Any surplus of vitamin A is stored in the liver, so most people have a good reserve. For good sources of the vitamin, see Table 7 on page 25.

B vitamins The RDA of an adult for vitamin B$_1$ is about 1mg. We can get about a third of this from 2oz (60g) of meat, bacon or heart, $1\frac{1}{2}$oz (45g) of peanuts or 2oz (60g) of oatmeal. Cereals are good sources of vitamin B$_1$. White bread in many countries is enriched with added vitamin

7 Good sources of vitamin A
Portions supplying one-third of RDA for an adult

Food (as preformed vitamin A or retinol)	Portion
Halibut-liver oil	1 drop (50mg)
Cod-liver oil	$\frac{1}{4}$teaspoon (1 g)
Liver (lamb and beef)	$\frac{1}{3}$oz (10g)
Liver (calf)	1oz (30g)
Butter (average)	1oz (30g)
Margarine	1oz (30g)
Eggs	2 eggs (100g)
Milk	$\frac{1}{2}$ pint (3dl)
Food *(as carotene)*	
Red palm-oil	$\frac{1}{6}$oz (5g)
Carrots (old)	$\frac{1}{3}$oz (10g)
Carrots (new, canned)	$\frac{2}{3}$oz (20g)
Spinach	$\frac{2}{3}$oz (20g)
Apricots (dried)	2oz (60g)
Watercress	$\frac{2}{3}$oz (20g)
Broccoli	$3\frac{1}{2}$oz (100g)
Tomatoes	2oz–1 lb (60–450g)
Corn	$2\frac{1}{4}$lb (1 kg)
Peppers (red)	$3\frac{1}{2}$oz (100g)
Peppers (green)	1 lb (450g)
Cabbage	10oz (300g)

B_1 so that 6oz (180g) of this, or 5oz (150g) of whole-grain bread will supply one-third of the daily B_1.

Vitamin B_2 is found in large supply in milk and liver— $\frac{2}{3}$ pint (4dl) of milk or $\frac{3}{4}$oz (20g) of liver will provide a third of the daily need, and there is some to be found also in tea and eggs.

Niacin is needed in a quantity of about 18mg a day. It is found in peanuts, bread, meat and coffee.

Yeast and yeast extract are very rich in vitamins B_1, B_2 and niacin. About $\frac{1}{2}$oz (15g) of brewer's yeast will supply one-third of the RDA.

Good sources of folic acid include liver, spinach and fish, and it is also found in green vegetables, whole-grain bread and eggs. Vitamin B_6 is widely distributed, but good sources include meat, especially liver, green vegetables and whole-grain bread.

Vitamin C The recommended daily intake of vitamin C is 60mg. It is commonly found in all fruit and vegetables, and Table 11 (page 28) shows that some are so rich in it that we could get all we need for a day from 4-5oz (110-140g) of grapefruit or orange, or as little as 1oz (30g) of peppers, black currants or parsley. Potatoes are unusual because while they are not a rich source of vitamin C they are

8 Good sources of niacin
Portions supplying one-third of RDA for an adult (6mg)

Food	Portion
Peanuts and peanut butter	1¾oz (50g)
Bread (whole-grain)	7oz (200g)
Yeast (baker's)	⅔oz (20g)
Yeast (brewer's)	½oz (15g)
Rice (white)	20oz (600g)
Rice (parboiled)	10oz (300g)
Soya flour	10oz (300g)
Meats	5oz (140g)
Mushrooms (dried)	3oz (90g)
Liver	2oz (60g)
Barley (pearled)	8oz (230g)
Coffee	⅓oz (10g)
Beer, mild	2 pints (1 liter)
Dried beans	10oz (300g)
Sunflower seed	3½oz (100g)
Yeast extract	⅓oz (10g)
Meat extract	½oz (15g)

9 Good sources of vitamin B₁
Portions supplying one-third of RDA for an adult (about 0.3mg)

Food	Portion
Heart (beef)	2oz (60g)
Bacon (lean)	2oz (60g)
Pork (lean)	1¾oz (50g)
Pork (fat)	2½oz (75g)
Cod's roe	¾oz (20g)
Liver and kidney	4oz (110g)
Dried beans	1½oz (45g)
Peanuts	1½oz (45g)
Potatoes	10oz (300g)
Oatmeal	2oz (60g)
Flour (whole-grain)	3oz (90g)
Flour (white, enriched)	4oz (110g)
Soya flour	½oz (15g)
Brazil nuts	1oz (30g)
Yeast (baker's)	½oz (15g)
Yeast (brewer's)	1/10oz (3g)
Bread (whole-grain)	5oz (140g)
Bread (white, enriched)	6oz (180g)
Bread (wheat germ)	¾oz (20g)

10 Good sources of vitamin B₂
Portions supplying one-third of RDA for an adult (about 0.5mg)

Food	Portion
Milk (cow's)	⅔ pint (4dl)
Hard cheese	3½oz (100g)
Liver	¾oz (20g)
Kidney	1oz (30g)
Tea (extract from leaves)	2oz (60g)
Skim-milk powder	1oz (30g)
Egg	5oz (140g)
Almonds	2½oz (75g)
Yeast (baker's)	1oz (30g)
Yeast (brewer's)	½oz (15g)
Soft curd-cheese	6oz (170g)

11 Sources of vitamin C
(Raw, edible portion, unless otherwise stated)

Food	mg/oz (30g)
Apples (eating, raw)	1
Bananas	3
Bean sprouts	8
Beetroot (cooked)	2
Black currants (raw)	56
Black currants (cooked or canned)	40
Breadfruit	6
Cabbage (raw)	18
Cabbages (cooked 5 mins)	6
Cabbages (cooked, kept hot 30 mins)	3
Gooseberries	12
Grapefruit juice (canned)	12
Grapefruit (whole)	5
Grapefruit (peeled, fresh)	12
Guava	56
Horseradish	34
Kale, broccoli, beet, greens, turnip tops	34
Leeks	6
Lemons (whole)	6
Lemons (juice)	12
Lettuce	4
Mango	8
Melon	8
Mustard greens	20
Okra	7
Oranges (whole)	10
Oranges (peeled)	15
Oranges (canned juice)	12
Parsley	44
Papaya	14
Peas (raw)	7
Peas (fresh, cooked)	4
Peas (canned, cooked)	3
Peas (dried by modern methods, cooked)	3
Peppers (green or red)	43

mg/100g	Portions supplying 25mg
4	1½lb (700g)—3 large apples
10	9oz (270g)
30	3oz (90g)
6	¾lb (340g)—1 large
200	½oz (15g)—½ tablespoon
140	¾oz (20g)—1 tablespoon
21	4oz (110g)
60	1½oz (45g)—1 cupful
20	5oz (140g)
10	8oz (230g)
40	2oz (60g)
42	2fl.oz (60ml)—wineglassful
17	5oz (140g)—½ small
42	2oz (60g)—8 sections
200	½oz (15g)
120	¾oz (20g)
120	¾oz (20g)
20	4oz (110g)
20	4oz (110g)—1 large
42	2fl.oz (60ml)—wineglassful
14	6oz (170g)—1 large
30	3oz (90g)
30	3oz (90g)
80	1oz (30g)
24	3½oz (100g)
35	2½oz (75g)—½ small orange
50	1½oz (45g)—4-5 sections
42	2fl.oz (60ml)—wineglassful
150	½oz (15g)
50	2oz (60g)
24	3½oz (100g)
15	6oz (170g)
10	8oz (230g)
10	8oz (230g)
150	½oz (15g)

continued on next page

Sources of vitamin C

continued from previous page
(Raw, edible portion, unless otherwise stated)

Food	mg/oz (30g)
Pineapple (fresh)	7
Pineapple (canned juice)	3
Plantain	6
Potatoes (new, cooked)	5
Potatoes (old, after January)	1
Red currants	12
Rosehip syrup	56
Rutabaga (cooked)	5
Scallions	7
Sprouts (raw)	28
Sprouts (cooked)	10
Strawberries	17
Sweet potato	8
Tomato (raw, cooked or juice)	7
Watercress	18
West Indian cherry	570
Yams (fresh)	3

eaten by the pound rather than the ounce and so supply a large proportion of the vitamin in the diet of many people. One of the problems, as discussed previously (pages 12-13), is that vitamin C can easily be lost in cooking-water and through numerous other factors, so it pays, in every respect, to be a careful cook.

Vitamin D Very few foods contain vitamin D and there is a possible shortage in children and adolescents who have a special need for bone growth, and in elderly people who are housebound and get little or no vitamin D from sunshine. The recommended intake is about 5-10 micrograms. The richest sources are fatty fish such as sardines, mackerel and pilchards, and it is added to margarine in many countries, to milk in the United States, and is also present in eggs, butter and liver. For good sources, see Table 12 on page 32.

Minerals

Absolute proof that our mineral intake is adequate is impossible, but just as with vitamins, anyone living on a Western diet is most unlikely to suffer from severe mineral-shortage leading to deficiency diseases. Again, the only way to ensure we are getting enough is to eat all

ng/100g)	Portions supplying 25mg
24	3½oz (100g)—1 slice ½in thick
10	½ pint (3dl)
21	4oz (110g)
18	5oz (140g)—2 med size
4	1½lb (700g)
40	2oz (60g)
200	½fl.oz (15ml)—2 teaspoons
18	5oz (140g)—large portion
25	3½oz (100g)
100	1oz (30g)—2-3 sprouts
35	2½oz (75g)—5-6 sprouts
60	1½oz (45g)
28	3oz (90g)
25	3-4oz (90-110g)—1-2 large tomatoes
60	1½oz (45g)
2000	1 small cherry
10	9oz (270g)

the right foods. However, if the diet is sufficiently varied so that it supplies enough iron, calcium, iodine, fluorine and zinc, it will almost certainly provide enough of all the other minerals needed.

Iron We can get one-third of our daily needs of iron from as little as 1oz (30g) of liver or kidney, or 3½oz (100g) of beef, or from 5oz (140g) of whole-grain bread or 8oz (230g) of enriched white bread. A teaspoon of curry powder, a tablespoon of cocoa or a tablespoon of molasses will also provide a third of the daily needs since they are rich sources, and most vegetables supply small amounts. The recommended daily intake is about 10-18mg. For good sources, see Table 13 on page 33.

Calcium We need about 1g of calcium a day. Portions of food that supply one-third of this would be 5fl.oz (140ml) fresh milk, between ½oz (15g) and 3½oz (100g) of cheese, depending on the type, and about 7oz (200g) of enriched white bread—there is little calcium in (unenriched) whole-grain bread.

One of the more unusual sources of calcium is the bones of fish. Some kinds, especially canned fish, are eaten with their bones and we could get one-third of our day's needs from as little as ⅓oz (10g) of some dried fish or 2oz (60g) of sardines. For good sources, see Table 14 on page 34.

Iodine and fluorine The main source of iodine is fish, and if fish is eaten once or twice a week there should be no deficiency. It may also be obtained from vegetables, milk and cereals, and it is usually possible to buy salt that has been enriched with iodine.

Fluorine is obtained mainly from drinking water, but there are also small amounts in food, especially fish, and tea. It is added to water in some places, although there appears to be a quite unreasonable opposition to such enrichment by some sections of the public.

Zinc There are traces of zinc in most foods, but good sources are whole-grain bread, hard cheeses, cocoa, meats, meat by-products, and shellfish, especially oysters.

12 Good sources of vitamin D
Portions supplying 1 μg

Food	Portion
Cod-liver oil	few drops (0.5g)
Fatty fish:	
Sprats	$\frac{1}{15}$oz (2g)
Herrings and kippers	$\frac{1}{6}$oz (5g)
Mackerel	$\frac{1}{6}$oz (5g)
Salmon (fresh or canned)	$\frac{1}{4}$oz (7g)
Sardines	$\frac{1}{2}$oz (15g)
Eggs	1oz (30g)—$\frac{1}{2}$ egg
Egg yolk	$\frac{1}{2}$oz (15g)
Margarine	$\frac{1}{2}$oz (15g)
Butter	5oz (140g)
Liver	3oz (90g)

Amounts supplying 20 μg of vitamin D

5 sprats	
2 herring filets	
2 kipper filets	
$\frac{1}{2}$oz (15g) eels	
2 teaspoons cod-liver oil	
1 small can of salmon	
4 eggs	
1 large can of sardines	
8oz (230g) margarine	

DIETARY FIBER

There is more to food than fats, proteins and other nutrients. For proper functioning of the intestine we need dietary fiber, or roughage. This is largely a type of carbohydrate material that cannot be digested and so passes along the digestive tract, giving the intestines something to work on.

13 Good sources of iron

Portions supplying one-third of RDA for an adult (4-5mg)

Food	Portion
Curry powder	⅙oz (5g)—1 teaspoon
Cocoa powder	1oz (30g)—1 heaped tablespoon
Baked beans	7oz (200g)—1 small can
Beans and peas (dry)	2½oz (75g)—half teacup
Lentils (dry)	2oz (60g)
Corned beef	1¼oz (35g)—1 slice
Liver or kidney	1oz (30g)—1 thin slice
Beef (cooked)	3½oz (100g)
Fish (fried)	12oz (340g)
Sardines	3½oz (100g)—1 small can
Oatmeal	3oz (90g)
Cornflakes, etc.	5oz (140g)
Almonds	3½oz (100g)
Heart	3oz (90g)
Soya flour	2oz (60g)—2 tablespoons
Shellfish	1¼oz (35g)
Molasses	1½oz (45g)—1 tablespoon
Bread (brown)	5oz (140g)
Bread (white)	8oz (230g)
Wheat germ	1¾oz (50g)
Green peas	8oz (230g)
Greens (cooked)	12oz (340g)
Greens (raw)	12oz (340g)
Yam and potatoes	12oz (340g)
Flour (white)	7oz (200g)
Flour (whole-grain)	4oz (110g)
Figs and apricots (dry)	3oz (90g)
Prunes (dry)	6oz (170g)
Pasta (dry)	10oz (300g)

14 Good sources of calcium
Portions supply about 200mg.

Food	Portion
Milk	½ pint (190ml)
Cheese	
Parmesan	½oz (15g)
Cheddar	1oz (30g)
Edam	1oz (30g)
Stilton	2oz (60g)
Whitebait (whole)	⅔oz (20g)
Sprats (whole)	1oz (30g)
Sardines	2oz (60g)
Pilchards (canned)	3oz (90g)
Soya beans	3oz (90g)
Tripe	5oz (140g)
Molasses	1½oz (45g)
Almonds	3oz (90g)
Kale	3oz (90g)
Broccoli	7oz (200g)
Beans	4oz (110g)
White bread (enriched)	8oz (230g)
White flour (enriched)	5oz (140g)
White flour (unenriched)	3lb (1⅓kg)

RDA for adults is 800mg, for children 1,200mg.

Fruit contains roughage as pectin, vegetables contain some as cellulose, but the most important and useful source is the bran of cereals, particularly in whole-grain cereals like whole-grain bread. Table 15 (page 36) shows principal sources of dietary fiber.

The value of roughage in the diet in helping to prevent constipation has been known (and ignored) for very many years, but recently a number of diseases growing more common in Western industrialized society have been linked with a shortage of roughage. We are eating much less bread, most of that is white (there is less fiber in white bread than in whole-grain), and the total amount of fiber in the diet is becoming less and less. Many people feel an immediate improvement in preventing constipation by eating bran as breakfast cereal, but other disorders that are not so obvious have been linked to a low-fiber diet. For example, it has been suggested that certain types of cancer of the intestine, varicose veins, heart disease and diabetes are linked with low-fiber diets, but this is not so easy to prove.

It is impossible to say just how much bran anyone should eat. Each person has to find out their own needs. If you are constipated, try taking three or four teaspoons of bran a day, increasing this to perhaps nine or ten teaspoons until the condition is alleviated. Remember that some of the bran breakfast cereals, which many people prefer to ordinary bran, have had sugar and flavor added, so you need about one and a half times as much as you would of ordinary bran.

Apart from bran itself, whole-grain bread is the best source of dietary fiber. Whole-grain bread is made from the whole wheat grain with all its bran: a slice of whole-grain bread is about equivalent to two teaspoons of bran. It is not the same to eat "brown" breads, which are usually partway between white and whole-grain; they may differ considerably in their bran content and will have much less than whole-grain bread.

A good idea would be to eat some whole-grain bread each day, take bran for breakfast and include it in recipes, and eat plenty of fruit and vegetables.

ARE WE PROPERLY FED?

Since the beginning of this century we have learned a great deal about vitamins, mineral salts and proteins, and we have a reasonable idea of how much the average person needs. We also have a very highly developed food industry, well-stocked supermarkets, cookbooks by the thousand and restaurants of all types. Are we all then properly nourished?

The answer is no, on two counts. Firstly, there is no guarantee that everyone is getting all the nutrients he or she needs, and secondly, there has been an enormous increase, in those very countries where these great food improvements have been taking place, in a whole range of diseases that seem to be connected with the diet. They are even called "diseases of affluence." They are due to many different factors, but diet does seem to be involved. They include heart disease, which has been increasing at an alarming rate over the past two generations in all industrialized communities; it seems that the richer people get, the "better" food they eat, but the more they worry about getting richer, the more deaths there are from heart disease. There have been similar increases in diseases of the bowel, including diverticulitis, cancer of the colon, and a group of related diseases. The same goes for obesity, dental decay and diabetes. Certainly some of these are partly inherited, but since it is now too late to change your parents, what can be done?

The rise in these disorders seems to have run parallel to an increased amount of fat in our diets. In many industrialized countries we now take between 40 and 45 percent of our energy from fats, and these are mostly animal fats in meat, milk, butter and cream. We have also

35

15 Principal sources of dietary fiber

Food	g/3½oz (100g)
Wheat bran	45
Wheat flour	3
Bread (whole-grain)	9
Bread (white)	3
Rice (boiled)	1
Cereal (cooked)	1
All Bran	27
Cornflakes	3
Muesli	about 7
Shredded Wheat	12
Mustard greens	4
Parsnips	4
Peas (garden)	5
Peas (processed)	8
Chickpeas (cooked)	6
Beans (snap)	3
Plantain (boiled)	6
Spinach (boiled)	6
Corn on the cob (boiled)	5
Apricots (stewed)	9
Blackberries (stewed)	6
Black currants (stewed)	7
Figs (dry)	20
Prunes (stewed)	8
Raisins	7
Raspberries	7
Potatoes	2
Potato chips	12

been increasing fats in ice cream, cakes and salad dressings. A high level of cholesterol in the blood, which has been shown to be a factor in atherosclerosis, is related to the amount and kind of fat in the diet. Fats, especially saturated fats in animal foods, increase the amount of cholesterol in the blood.

We have also increased our sugar until it amounts to a fifth of the total food-intake (that is an average; some eat far more sugar than this), and we have been eating less and less food that contains any form of dietary fiber.

A SENSIBLE APPROACH

Obviously we cannot go through life selecting and weighing out the foods listed in the tables—it would cause havoc in a restaurant and offend any hostess. How then can we try to make sure that we eat the right foods in sufficient quantity to get all the nutrients we need?

The first point to bear in mind is that if you eat a wide variety of foods there is more chance of your obtaining all the different nutrients. This may sound elementary, because most people eat a varied diet just because they like different food, but there are some people who live on a very monotonous and restricted diet who may well develop shortages of some nutrients.

The second point is to avoid diluting the diet with "empty calories": reduce sugar and sweet foods, reduce fats and oils, and keep alcoholic drinks down to a reasonable level (see ALCOHOL, pages 40-42). There is certainly nothing wrong with an occasional large helping of cake, dessert or fatty foods, or with an occasional drink—unless, of course, you are trying to lose weight (see OBESITY AND DIETING, pages 53-61).

DIETARY GOALS

Nutritionists recommend up to six basic dietary modifications that they consider desirable for good health. These are: if you are overweight, lose the excess; eat less fat; eat less sugar; take more dietary fiber; take less salt; and moderate your alcohol intake. Dietary changes such as these cannot do us any harm, and are likely (although, of course, not by any means certain) to reduce the risk of heart disease and bowel complaints, and possibly also of stroke, blood pressure, and other disorders.

How to set about it

You can hardly be expected to change your eating habits overnight. After all, it took a lifetime to acquire them, and you can expect to need some time to change them.

You may find it easier to tackle it in stages: gradually take a little less sugar in your tea and coffee, eat fewer candies and sweet food, buy leaner meat, have less fat on your bread, change to brown bread, use less salt and salty foods, and eat more fruit and vegetables.

You should be aiming to get by with a little less rather than setting yourself a target of *never* eating *any* of the "less healthy" foods. Even dieters are "allowed" the occasional half a chocolate éclair or a small glass of wine. "Moderation in all things" should be the rule—even in improving your eating habits.

What it all means

Lose weight The dangers of overweight, recommendations for how to lose it and methods of prevention are discussed in OBESITY AND DIETING (pages 53-61). Many illnesses are made more serious by overweight even if they do not result directly from obesity. A prime requirement for better health, then, is to maintain your correct weight.

Less fat It may never be proved that "too much" fat is a prime cause of many modern diseases, but it is generally accepted that we would all benefit from taking less fat.

But how much is "too much"? The *Report of the US Senate Select Committee on Nutrition and Human Needs* (1977) stated that fat supplied approximately 40 percent of the total energy of the average US diet. It recommended that this should be reduced to about 30 percent. Many authorities in other countries have made similar recommendations ranging between 30 and 35 percent.

The reason for this advice is that it has been established that a high intake of fats, particularly of the saturated fats from animal foods, increases the level of cholesterol in the blood. Since high levels of blood cholesterol are considered to be a risk factor in heart disease a reduction in fat-consumption should be beneficial. Saturated fats, the worst offenders, are present in meat and milk, and so in butter and cream.

Some vegetable oils contain polyunsaturates that can reduce the blood cholesterol-level, and it is therefore a good idea to substitute polyunsaturates (as in the special margarines and cooking oils) for saturated fats. But avoid simply adding extra polyunsaturates to your diet—the aim, after all, is to eat altogether less fat.

Less sugar Sugar has been blamed for numerous problems, ranging from obesity and dental decay to diabetes and heart disease. Although none of this is scientifically proved, authorities advise taking less sugar: you should aim to reduce it by half.

The strongest criticism of sugar is that it contains only "empty calories." This means that sugar provides only energy without any nutrients, unlike other foods such as bread, potatoes, fruits and vegetables which supply protein, vitamins and minerals as well as energy.

More dietary fiber Constipation and possibly many other bowel disorders are helped by extra dietary fiber. It comes from whole-grain cereals, for which the chief source is whole-grain bread, and a significant amount is found even in milled cereals and white bread, as well as in all kinds of fruits and vegetables.

Nutritionists recommend a 50-percent increase in dietary fiber. Part of this can be achieved by taking a bran preparation, but some people whose systems cannot tolerate bran may need instead a medicinal form of fiber.

For anyone suffering from constipation there is no actual prescribed "dose" of bran. Each person has to find how much he or she needs. Start with half a dozen teaspoons of bran a day and gradually increase this amount until the problem disappears. You should also eat more potatoes, bread, root crops, fruit and vegetables as sources of fiber to make up for eating less fat and sugar.

Less salt We all take five to ten times more salt than we really need. Although it is still debated whether there is positively any benefit from taking less salt, it seems that it cannot actually cause any harm. Our food already contains enough natural salt to which we add more during cooking and often even more at the table. Moreover, many manufactured foods contain salt. So there is clearly ample scope for reducing our salt intake.

Moderate alcohol Nutritionists seem to keep telling us what is bad for us, so it may be a relief to be told that alcohol—in moderation, of course—is actually beneficial. It helps in promoting healthy blood-flow and to some extent in preventing the formation of blood clots (thrombosis) caused by weakness of the blood platelets.

Excessive alcohol, on the other hand, is harmful because it damages the liver and brain; in the long run it is a killer. Guidelines are provided in Table 16—although (at least some) women may be disappointed to learn that their "ration" is smaller than that of men.

16 Moderate amounts of alcohol

	Alcohol	Spirits		Wine		Beer
	gm	ml	fl.oz	ml	fl.oz	
Men	34	100	3½	340	12	2 pints (1 liter)
Women	23	70	2½	230	8	1¼ pints (700ml)

Excessive amounts

Men	80	240	8½	800	28	4 pints (2 liters)
Women	50	160	5½	500	20	2¾ pints (1½ liters)

WHAT ABOUT CHOLESTEROL?

In the *Report of the US Senate Select Committee on Nutrition and Human Needs* it was stated that the average US citizen ingests 600 mg of cholesterol a day, "well above the 400-mg limit which has a direct effect on the blood cholesterol-levels."

Although some medical authorities place less importance upon the effect of dietary cholesterol on the levels of cholesterol in the blood, most of them agree with the recommendation of the Senate committee that dietary cholesterol should be reduced to 300 mg or less a day.

Alcohol

From the earliest days man discovered how to ferment carbohydrates with yeast and so make alcohol. When we talk about alcohol as a drink we always mean ethyl alcohol, but some people have poisoned themselves by drinking methyl alcohol, also called wood spirit. Around the world there are many different varieties of drinks—even fermented milk such as kumiss and kefir—but most of them fall into one of three groups: beer, wines, or spirits (hard liquor).

They differ mainly in their alcoholic content—as any-

17 Nutritional value of alcoholic drinks

	Alcohol (%)	Sugar (%)
Lager	2.6	1.6
Mild beer	2.6	1.6
Stout (bottled)	2.9	4.2
Cider (dry, fermented)	3.8	2.6
Cider (sweet, fermented)	3.8	4.3
Wine (red/white)	9.0	0.3
Wine (sweet)	10.0	6.0
Port	16.0	12.0
Sherry	16.0	1–7
Spirits	30.0	0
Cherry brandy	19.0	30
Curacao	30.0	30

18 Nutritional value of soft drinks

	Sugar (%)
Cokes	10
Grapefruit or orange juice (unsweetened)	8
Grapefruit or orange juice (sweetened)	10
Pineapple juice	13
Lemonade (bottled)	6
Tomato juice	3
Fruit drinks (diluted with 4 parts water)	6

one knows when drinking beer by the pint, wine by the glass and spirits in smaller glasses. Beer, ale and stout are mostly 2-3-percent alcohol together with some carbohydrate (except in beer made specially for diabetics). Wines are mostly 9-10-percent alcohol but may contain 8-13 percent depending on how much sugar there was in the grapes. The alcohol content, however, cannot go much above 13 percent even when sugar is added to the fruit, because the alcohol kills off the yeast. Sherry and port are fortified by adding brandy and so are about 15-percent alcohol. Spirits such as brandy, whiskey and gin are 30-percent alcohol, which is about as strong a solution of alcohol as the mouth can stand. They are made by distilling the alcohol from wine and then diluting it.

In some countries the alcohol content is labeled as

Energy per 3½ fl. oz (100ml)		Energy per pint (½ liter)	
Cal	kJ	Cal	kJ
25	104	125	520
25	104	140	600
40	160	200	800
35	150	200	870
40	170	240	1000
70	290		
90	400		

Energy per 2 fl. oz (60ml)	
90	400
70	290
130	550
150	630
190	800

Energy per 3½ fl. oz (100ml)		Energy per 7 fl. oz (200ml)	
Cal	kJ	Cal	kJ
40	170	80	340
30	130	60	260
40	170	80	350
50	220	100	440
20	80	40	170
15	70	30	140
20	80	40	170

"degrees proof" spirit instead of by percentage. "Proof spirit" in the UK is 57 percent alcohol by volume and in the USA it is 50 percent. So pure alcohol is 175 degrees proof in the UK and 200 degrees proof in the USA. This is why the same bottle of whiskey can be labeled 70 degrees proof (UK) and 84 degrees proof (USA).

"Proof spirit" was a term invented before chemists were as skilled as they are today. It is the strength of alcohol that will ignite when mixed with gunpowder. In the old days, that was when we paid tax; now the chemists are more skilled we pay tax on all alcoholic drinks.

There is no doubt that alcohol is a chemical that is foreign to our bodies, that it is a poison, and that regular, excessive drinking is harmful and can lead to chronic alcoholism. But few people suffer any harm from taking alcoholic drinks in moderation. Social drinking "lifts the spirit, loosens the tongue and removes the inhibitions, so enhancing social intercourse"—and general enjoyment.

Table 17 (pages 40-41) shows several categories of alcoholic drink.

Alcohol has very little nutritional value. Spirits provide nothing but energy. Beer does supply a reasonable amount of two of the B vitamins: between 1.5 and 4mg niacin per pint ($\frac{1}{2}$ liter), depending on the strength, which is 10-20 percent of the RDA, and also about 10-20 percent of the RDA of vitamin B_2.

Wines have no more than mere traces of vitamins, but they do contain some iron: a wine glass ($3\frac{1}{2}$ fl. oz or 100ml) will supply about 1mg of iron, which is 10 percent of the RDA; and the iron in wine appears to be well absorbed. Thus if you drink you would do better to stick to beer or wine—getting some nutrients along with the calories.

You can work out from Table 17 that two glasses of whiskey (with or without soda) before a meal, three glasses of wine during it and a glass of liqueur afterwards will give you, in round figures, 650 Calories (2,500 kilojoules)—about as much as a small meal.

There is evidence that alcohol taken in moderation helps blood circulation and strengthens the blood platelets. These are small cells that help the blood to clot when bleeding occurs, but if they break down too easily they can cause blood clots, or thrombosis, in the arteries. So moderate amounts of alcohol can be actually helpful.

The problem is to decide just how much is "moderate." It is well established that, leaving aside the social consequences, too much alcohol can lead to heart disease, can damage the liver and brain, and, long-term, is often fatal.

A recent recommendation came from the committee advising the UK Department of Health. While not saying that alcohol is actually beneficial, the committee reported that a certain amount can be taken with safety. General guidelines on "moderate" amounts of alcohol are provided in Table 16 on page 39.

Fresh or processed food?

BETTER OR WORSE?

Many people who are concerned about their diets will look for fresh rather than processed food. Are they right? The answer is that some fresh foods are better than processed foods, some are worse and others are the same.

Firstly, it must be kept in mind that some losses are intentional, such as when vegetables are trimmed, or fish eviscerated, or foodstuffs such as olive oil or sugar are extracted from the olive or the sugar cane, or when wheat is milled to white flour. The part that is lost is unwanted.

Secondly, cooking is itself a process that causes inevitable losses. Heat always destroys some small part of the nutrients, and severe heat, such as in roasting and baking, causes greater losses. Some part of the water-soluble nutrients, particularly vitamin C in fruit and vegetables, and vitamin B_1 in meat, is washed out into the cooking water, but they are saved, of course, if the cooking juices are consumed.

Thirdly, a lot of our manufactured foods are canned or bottled and come to us ready-cooked. Any losses that may take place in the factory are then *instead* of those that would inevitably take place in our own kitchens, not *additional* to them. By the time the foods reach our plates they probably do not differ much in nutritional content whether they were processed in the factory or cooked at home. So much depends on how fresh the food was to start with, how good the cook is compared with the factory, and whether we really prefer maximum nutritional content to good taste. The very nice taste of roast meat is due largely to damaged protein, but nobody is going to say that roasting should be banned. In any case, the losses are small and anyone who eats meat is not going to suffer from protein shortage.

Then there is the question of what is meant by "fresh foods." They can be garden-fresh, meaning just-harvested, or market-fresh, meaning that a week or more may have passed since they were harvested. Generally the manufacturer starts with garden-fresh food, while the home cook may have to put up with vegetables that are rather stale and tired. Frozen fish is often frozen and even cooked at sea within hours of being caught, while "fresh" fish in the fishmarket may be 2-3 weeks old.

Generally speaking it is vitamin C that suffers most in cooking and processing, and to a lesser extent vitamin B_1 in some foods; there is also a small loss in the quality of the protein. Garden-fresh foods are the best, frozen foods next best, then canned foods; dried foods, on average, probably are least good. But the main loss is of vitamin C—there is no need to worry about the other nutrients.

Balancing losses against advantages

The main advantage of processing foods is that they are preserved (by canning, freezing, salting or drying) and will then keep for months or years. It means we can get foods all year around and from all countries. So even if processing does cause some loss of nutrients, at least we do get the food. In fact, it would be quite impossible without food-processing to feed the large numbers of people living in cities; so in some cases it is not a question of processed food versus fresh food, but processed food versus no food whatever.

There are also health advantages, such as in the pasteurization of milk. Although pasteurization destroys about a quarter of the vitamin C in milk and a tenth of the vitamins B_1, B_6, B_{12} and folic acid, this is a price worth paying for the safety from disease that can occur from drinking raw, untreated milk. More modern methods, such as selling sterilized milk in cardboard containers, suffer about the same loss but make milk available to many people, especially children, who would not otherwise get any.

Certainly not all food manufacturers pay attention to the nutritional value of their products, and many processed foods could be of higher nutritional quality if they were more carefully made or better methods of processing were used. At the same time, not all cooks are angels in the kitchen: some of them damage both the nutritional quality and the taste of foods far more than any manufacturer would ever dare do, for he would not be able to sell the products that are inflicted on some families.

SOME MYTHS

The recent interest in food and health has given rise to numerous articles in the press, and radio and television programs, not all of which present the facts correctly. This publicity has given rise to several modern myths.

Convenience foods These are blamed for many, if not all, of our modern ills, from dental decay and obesity to constipation and cancer. In fact, convenience foods, as such, are not to blame for anything, because the term simply means foods that have been partly or largely prepared for us by the manufacturer.

Bread was one of the earliest convenience foods. The manufacturer saves us the trouble of making it ourselves, it can be used for many purposes, it is easily carried about and keeps fairly well. In fact, whole-grain bread is generally regarded as being a very "healthy" food. When wheat is milled to white flour to make the white bread that many people prefer, part of the nutrients are lost—but that is a different matter.

In the same way, anything canned or bottled is ready to eat without further preparation apart perhaps from warming. Such convenience foods can be, although they are not always, as good as the same foods cooked at home; depending on the cook, they can taste better or worse, and can be nutritionally better or worse, than those made at home. Each food and each process would have to be considered individually.

Fast foods Technically-speaking these are foods that can be prepared quickly on a large scale, and retail outlets therefore specialize in only a few foods instead of offering the larger menu which one expects in a restaurant. An early version of these fast-food outlets was the old fish-fish-and-chip shop (French fries), followed later by shops specially selling chicken, pizzas or hamburgers.

As regards nutrients, they are similar to the same thing produced at home; after all, a hamburger is only chopped-up meat. The criticism often made of hamburgers and some other fast-food products is that they are relatively rich in fat and salt. What we do not know is whether they contain more fat and salt than would the same dish prepared at home; presumably, if customers demanded, they could be "improved" in this respect.

In any manufactured product, of course, cheaper ingredients may be used. For example, it is most unlikely that any manufactured fish cake will contain as much fish as a housewife would use, simply because it would cost too much. In the same way, a meat product might contain more fat, or a fish finger more batter or breadcrumbs, than the equivalent food made at home. On the other hand, some people prefer their fish with batter....

Junk foods This is a term that has been applied to any food which is considered by the particular speaker or writer to be inferior. Scientifically the term means foods that supply energy and very little else; sugar and candies supply energy without any nutrients, but any food in which the sugar content is high and the nutrients proportionately low would fall into this class.

The American *World Book Dictionary*, on the other hand, defines junk food as: "Ready-made or quickly prepared food, as that available in vending machines and fast-food establishments." The term "junk food," then, seems to have become a derogatory term—yet the nutritional value and taste of such foods can be, and often is, as good as that which "mother makes"; and if mother is a poor cook, they can be better.

Frozen foods These are subjected to much less treatment than any other process except for simple chilling or refrigeration. The freezing process itself and subsequent storage have no ultimate effect on nutritional value, but they have to be preceded by a blanching process—a few minutes' hot-water treatment—to destroy the enzymes naturally present, which would otherwise continue to function during frozen storage and thus spoil the food. This short cooking process washes out a small amount (depending on the size of the pieces of food) of the water-soluble nutrients, of which only vitamin C is of any importance.

However, since frozen foods are already partly cooked, they need less cooking at home than fresh foods do, and the combined effect of processing and shorter cooking time has been shown to be about the same as the longer cooking needed for fresh foods.

There is no nutritional change during frozen storage provided temperature is kept down to $0°F$ ($-18°C$), but there can be a further loss while the food is being thawed. But because the manufacturer almost always starts with fresher fruits and vegetables than the housewife can obtain from the shops, and because these therefore contain more vitamin C, frozen meals can actually have more vitamin C than a freshly cooked meal.

Microwave cooking Microwave cookers make use of electromagnetic radiation which quickly generates heat throughout the bulk of the food. This contrasts with conventional cooking where heat is applied to the surface of the food and has to be conducted into the inner parts.

The term "radiation"—although heat is itself infrared radiation—sometimes causes concern about microwave cooking. There is absolutely no cause for worry unless the cooker itself is in such poor condition that the door fits badly so that radiation can leak out.

Irradiation The latest technique for treating food is by ionizing irradiation, of the same type as X-ray. Although the process sounds dangerous because the radiation usually comes from radioactive cobalt, it is in no way harmful. A food cooked in an electric oven is hardly likely to electrocute the consumer; it is equally wrong to suppose that ionizing radiation will make the food itself radioactive. The process has been thoroughly investigated for more than 20 years and internationally declared safe.

It has proved to be of value in eliminating the hazard of food-poisoning, by destroying the bacteria without affecting the food itself. It is particularly useful in preventing salmonella-poisoning from frozen poultry, which is an extremely common problem. Small doses kill off insects that infest stored grain, prevent fruits and vegetables from going moldy, and prevent stored potatoes from sprouting.

It is therefore a most useful innovation. Yet surprisingly there is nothing new about this "latest" advance. X-rays were discovered in 1895, and as long ago as 1896 it was suggested that irradiation could be used to destroy bacteria in food. The process itself was patented half a century ago, but it is only now being permitted in a large number of countries.

Health foods and special diets

The term "health foods" is popularly applied to a large variety of foods and dietary practices, ranging from ones of excellent nutritional quality to ones which at best are of very doubtful value. Some practical preoccupations of "health food" adherents are discussed below.

"NATURAL" FOODS

In recent years many people, especially town dwellers, have found great pleasure—and fresh food—in growing their own crops. This has led to exaggerated claims for anything that is "natural," a fact that advertisers have not been slow to spot. We even have the ludicrous situation where margarine is advertised as being made from natural oils in opposition to claims that butter is natural. Natural vitamins—those extracted from foods—are more highly prized and consequently more highly priced than those made in a factory. In fact, the synthetic vitamin has to be identical in all respects with the natural one and possesses all its biological functions.

CHEMICAL ADDITIVES

As discussed earlier, the greater part of all our food is processed; almost the only foods that we eat fresh are some fruits and vegetables at certain seasons of the year. Processing includes the addition of a large number of chemicals as preservatives, for coloring, flavoring and many other purposes. Ready-peeled potatoes, for instance, are dipped into a solution of bisulphite to keep them from going brown, and this destroys some of their vitamin B_1—the price you pay for convenience. Sausages are preserved with sulphur dioxide as a safety measure in some countries, including the UK, and this destroys all the vitamin B_1, but this must be balanced against the possible health risk of untreated sausages.

Certainly colors are added to food for purely cosmetic reasons. This is what most people seem to want. Butter is colored in some states to standardize the color all year around, and so are fruit-juice drinks. The consumer has now been conditioned to believe that pale orange drinks must be low in fruit-juice content, that the gray color of canned garden peas makes them unpalatable, and that the brown color of undyed strawberry jam is a mark of an inferior product.

There is currently no evidence that these additives do any harm, but neither is there evidence that they are

47

perfectly safe. Some of the colorings used in foods are derived from plants and there is a tendency to assume that this makes them safer than the synthetic ones. In fact, this is quite incorrect. There are plenty of poisonous substances in nature and the natural additives are just as open to suspicion as any invented by man.

HOMEMADE FOODS

Health-food shops often stock homemade products in preference to factory-made ones. For example, many people like to buy homemade, hand-potted jam, which sometimes makes the additional claim of being cooked in copper pots. The appeal, of course, is a nostalgic one, for there is no reason at all for hand-potted jam to be superior to jam that enters the pot through a machine-controlled tap or valve—in fact, the factory jam may be potted more hygienically. Moreover, boiling the jam in copper pots destroys vitamin C very rapidly, while boiling in stainless steel does not.

On the other hand, if you make jam or marmalade yourself you may very well end up with a better product than a factory-made one. Most cooks can make jam, and certainly marmalade, that will set by using only fruit and sugar, whereas the commercial products are usually diluted with extra sugar because it is cheaper than fruit pulp and so need to have extra pectin added to make them set. So if the list of ingredients on the label includes pectin, it means that less fruit has been used and more sugar has been added. In fact many of the health-food, homemade, high-priced jams and marmalades also contain extra pectin, so there is no reason to assume that these are richer in fruit than the factory products.

Although extra fruit may make a great deal of difference to the taste it will make very little difference to nutritional value, providing only a little extra vitamin C.

A cake which you have made yourself might be nutritionally superior to a factory product, because the manufacturer would use, say, fewer eggs and less milk to keep prices down. But unless you know what has gone into a product, you cannot assume that the label "homemade" on produce in health-food shops guarantees that it has more value than factory produce.

"WHOLE FOODS"

Some health foods are described as "whole foods," meaning that they are unrefined or that no more has been removed from the plant than is necessary to make it edible. The foods in question are mainly cereal grains and brown sugar (although it should be noted that the outer part of oat bran, which has been used to polish metal, is not well tolerated by the human digestive tract). Whole wheat and rice are certainly nutritionally preferable to white flour and polished rice, since they are richer in vitamins and iron, and very much richer in dietary fiber. Brown sugar, on the other hand, differs very little from white in its nutritional value. White sugar is 99.9-percent pure sucrose; brown 98-percent pure sucrose and 1-percent water; only the remaining 1 percent contains traces (but only traces) of vitamins and minerals. Molasses is a little less refined, but even so it contains only iron in any reasonable amount.

ORGANICALLY GROWN FOOD

While choosing to eat unprocessed or whole-grain foods creates no problems for other people, a widespread insistence on organically grown food would limit the amount of food that could be produced.

There is no evidence whatsoever that plants grown on soil organically manured by vegetable compost and animal droppings, and animals fed on such plants, are superior to those grown with or nourished on food grown with the aid of inorganic fertilizers such as sulphate of ammonia, phosphate and potash. In fact inorganic fertilizers are the *natural* food for plants, which take in their nutrients from the soil in the inorganic form supplied by nitrates, potassium salts and phosphates, and the trace elements. If, instead, they are supplied from an organic source such as rotted garden compost, animal manure, blood meal or hoof-and-horn meal (all of which are used by many gardeners) they must first be broken down in the soil to the relevant inorganic form before they can be absorbed by the plants.

It is true that organic material improves the texture and water-holding properties of the soil and that its nutrients are steadily released, but the latter can also be achieved by slow-release inorganic fertilizers. The best methods of cultivation would probably involve both organic and inorganic fertilizers, but this can be achieved only on a small scale. There is simply not enough organic material available to fertilize the vast areas of land needed to feed millions of people. If we did without inorganic fertilizers we would not produce enough food.

It is also argued that tractors compress the soil, that drips of tractor oil and fuel kill off earthworms, and that such ill-managed soil is less productive than organically manured soil untouched by the dead weight of a tractor. Even if this were true, it is difficult to visualize without these mechanical aids the vast Canadian wheatlands or the enormous areas in the USA where soya beans and corn are produced on such a gigantic scale that they feed populations around the world.

The same is true of the insecticides, herbicides and fungicides that are used on a vast scale in an attempt—not always successful—to protect crops from all their predators. Some have been pressed into use before being proved safe; but most countries now control the types of chemicals used and apply a limit to the amounts of such chemicals that may be left residually in the food. Studies of our food have shown that the levels are very low, but obviously it would be preferable if they were nonexistent. Unfortunately, this would once again severely curtail the amount of food produced.

VITAMIN SUPPLEMENTS

If you are getting enough vitamins in your diet, a supplement is not going to make you any healthier. There is no evidence to support the claims made for taking huge doses of vitamins ("megavitamin theory")—indeed, we know that vitamins A and D are toxic in large quantities. It may, however, be a good idea, and it will certainly do no harm, to take a small supplement (2 or 3 tablets of mixed vitamins a week) just in case your diet is deficient.

"MAGIC FOODS"

This category of health foods is a source of nonsense and profiteering. It sometimes seems that the principle is that a food is very good for you provided it is rarely eaten in your country. For example, buckwheat is almost unknown in the UK apart from in pet-food shops, but it is highly regarded by some health-food devotees. In Canada and the USA it is an ordinary vegetable, so commonly eaten that there is little point in making a specialty of it, and in central Europe it is the food of the peasants. That may make it very ordinary or very special, depending on your point of view.

Similarly, when yogurt was little known in the West it gained a special esteem. There were stories of Balkan peasants who lived to the magical age of 107 through eating it. Now that yogurt has become a very common food it has lost its "magical" properties—unless, of course, it is "live" yogurt instead of pasteurized "dead" material; then it regains its properties, we are told.

Honey occupies a special place in food mythology, possibly because of its unique source and because it has been known for so many thousands of years. It has been claimed to cure a multitude of disorders from tiredness to baldness, to secure sexual virility and to confer tallness. In fact it is simply a solution of sugars (glucose and fructose) together with a very small trace of some vitamins and minerals—not enough to make it into a reasonable food even if eaten in large quantities. It has an attractive taste, depending on the flowers that the bees browsed on, but it has no special properties that sugar—white sugar at that—does not have.

Seaweed, especially kelp, is sold in health-food shops as particularly beneficial, although there is not a trace of evidence that it has any value other than as a source of iodine. Sea salt, which contains iodine but also traces of all the impurities of seawater, is sold at a very much higher price than the pure salt obtained on land.

Another delightful oddity is bee's royal jelly, once well described as "this b... nonsense." It is claimed to have rejuvenating qualities, and so instantly appeals to all of us who cannot otherwise prevent ourselves growing older—so long as we can afford the extremely high price. Since this is the food that transforms a worker bee into a queen bee, it must clearly be very good for human beings. The only problem—glossed over in the claims—is that a bee is very small: if you multiply the bee's dose by the relative weight of an adult you would need to eat 20 tons a day—assuming that you wanted to be transformed into a queen bee.

PILLS AND POTIONS

Products for sale in health-food shops often include pills, potions, and sometimes even charms with far-reaching and untenable claims. These products are sometimes made from herbs and flowers that have been thought over the centuries to be beneficial for some disorders, but there is no evidence that they have any effect whatever—except, maybe, through faith in them. Such products are often bought in the same way that lucky charms or witches' blessings were bought centuries ago—and if people believe that something will do them good it may actually help them.

Among the "cures" are simple salts that, taken in the "right" combination, alleviate, if they do not cure, aches, pains, discharges of the ears, and a host of other disorders. You may wonder why people should pay for tablets made from simple salts, but the answer is that they are not described in simple terms. For example, everyone knows that table salt is cheap and available in every kitchen, and many people know that the chemical name is sodium chloride, but very few know that the old name is natrium muriate. So people pay good money for "natrium muriate" without knowing that they are already consuming more of this than is good for them. Similarly, no one would pay for sand (except to mix with cement), but call it "silicon dioxide" and it assumes a special function. So does plaster of Paris when called "calcium sulphate."

Such "cures" are not merely misleading but can also be dangerous, since their existence suggests that self-treatment is preferable to taking medical advice.

VEGETARIANISM

Meat-eaters tend to believe that meat is essential for "strength" and that one cannot live without it. This is not true; in fact, in some respects, a vegetarian is eating a better diet than a meat-eater. If, as discussed earlier, one of the errors of our Western diets is that we eat too much saturated fat, then the vegetarian is eating a better diet, since most of our saturated fat comes from meat. Again, dietary fiber is beneficial, and most vegetarians are eating whole-grain cereals, which contain a great deal of dietary fiber. Finally, as already pointed out, it is a good idea to eat a wide variety of foods in order to make sure of getting all the nutrients that we need; because vegetarians are more interested in diet than most people they do tend to eat a wider variety of foods, especially of fruits, vegetables, nuts and legumes, even if their diet is restricted by losing out on the nutrients present in meat, poultry and fish.

So far as we know, the health of vegetarians is as good as that of most other people. They would claim that it is better.

Meat is certainly an excellent source of protein, of iron that is well absorbed and of a range of vitamins of the B group, but there are plenty of people in the world living, by necessity if not from choice, on a vegetarian diet.

VEGANISM

A vegan diet excludes anything that comes from an animal, so milk, eggs, butter and cheese are not eaten, nor is meat, fish and poultry. Vegans appear to maintain good health on their diet, but it is much more difficult to follow than vegetarianism and its success depends on knowing a fair amount about nutrition.

MACROBIOTIC DIET

Among the more esoteric diets is the Zen macrobiotic diet, which originated in the USA and is concerned with spiritual awakening or rebirth. It has been publicly criticized by the American Medical Association, firstly because the diet is supposed to replace all medical treatment and, secondly, because as the stages of the diet progress it becomes increasingly restricted and there is therefore the danger of incurring serious nutritional deficiencies. There have been many victims of such deficiencies and even some deaths caused by this diet in the USA.

Obesity and dieting

One of the most common, most talked about and most ignored problems of nutrition is obesity—most common because a quarter to a third (some reports say half) of the population of all industrialized countries is overweight; most talked about and most ignored because obese people tend to talk about their problem but do little else.

CAUSES OF OBESITY

We don't really know the true cause of obesity, but we do know that anyone gaining weight is eating more food energy than he or she is using up in activity. That is a simple statement of fact. What we do not know is why some people eat more food than they use up and why some people can eat large quantities without getting fat.

Earlier, Table 3 (page 18) showed a balance sheet for an office worker who consumed 2,620 Calories (11 megajoules) per day as food and spent about the same amount of energy in activity, so maintaining constant weight. If his body functioned mechanically (and in this sense some people's bodies do) and he ate one more slice of bread and butter a day, he would gain weight. A slice of bread and butter provides about 100 Calories (420 kilojoules) per day, which would about to 10 lb (4.5 kg) of fat in a year. If this happened between the ages of 20 and 40 the extra daily slice of bread and butter could make him gain 200 lb (90 kg): he would at the age of 40 weigh 2½ times what he weighed at twenty.

How then is it that at least half the population do not gain or lose weight? Can they really eat exactly the amount of energy they use? The fat office worker ate only 100 Calories (420 kilojoules) extra per day, and gained 200 lb (90 kg); if he ate 10 Calories (42 kilojoules) extra he would, at the same rate, gain 20 lb (9 kg). Ten Calories (42 kilojoules) is one-tenth of a slice of bread and butter, or a few crumbs at each meal. Do people who maintain constant body weight really control their appetites to within a few crumbs a day?

The answer seems to be that some people, the ones whose weight stays the same for years on end, adjust their energy output to match their food intake, not the other way around. In other words, they burn off any surplus they have eaten, while their less fortunate friends are much more efficient and keep, as fat, all the extra food they eat. Some people appear to function like a savings bank—energy in minus energy out equals gain (or loss) of weight. Others are apparently born with a different mechanism, and whatever they eat they somehow keep their weight constant.

Then there are people who really do eat greedily, never leaving the table while there is food still on it. Most of these people will get fat, but why do they behave in this way? The behavioral scientists have been looking closely at such people during the last few years and conclude that they "eat with their eyes." The sight of food appears to act as a trigger to make them feel hungry; when they don't see it they don't feel hungry. The appetite of more "normal" people does not depend on seeing food.

People who say, "Why can she eat [it is usually she] twice as much as me and stay as skinny as a rail while I eat very little and every ounce stays on?" are sometimes not being quite truthful about their own eating habits. However, it is true that some people are born with small requirements; that is, a low metabolic rate. The average adult man, for example, who is moderately active eats about 2,500-3,000 Calories (10-12 megajoules) a day. If his weight does not change he must be using this amount. But some men of the same size and age, and doing the same work, may need only 2,000 Calories (8 megajoules), and so would get fat on a diet of 3,000 Calories (12 megajoules). Yet others need 4,000 Calories (16 megajoules): people really do differ as much as this, and even more. So a person with a lower metabolic rate (meaning simply that he or she burns off energy at a lower rate) will get fat even by eating only normal portions of food.

HOW FAT IS TOO FAT?

Despite all these different factors it is still true that anyone gaining weight is taking in more than they are using, and anyone who is currently fat must have done that at some time. But how fat is "fat"—and what is "excess weight"?

Firstly, it is fat, or adipose tissue, that we are really talking about, not weight. People can be heavier than average, but not fat, if they develop large muscles. Weight, however, is almost always a useful guide to body fat.

Secondly, people differ a great deal from one another in every respect, including their "ideal" body-weight, but the best we can do is to compare them with the *average* weight. It has been shown by insurance company statistics that people of average body-weight, or slightly less, live longer than those who are 12lb (6kg) or more above average weight. The heavier you are the shorter life you can expect. Men who are 10-percent overweight have a 13-percent increased death risk. This rises to 25 percent if they are 20-percent overweight and to 42 percent if they are 30-percent overweight. For women the increased death risk is 9 percent, 21 percent and 30 percent for each of the stages of fatness.

Put another way, a man over 45 who is 25lb (12kg) overweight reduces his life expectancy by 25 percent: he is likely to die at 60 instead of 80. Studies have shown that if he loses his surplus fat he greatly reduces the risk. These, of course, are averages; some fat people live a long time (and some thin people die young).

Fat people have increased risk of diabetes, and high blood pressure with the many disorders that this gives rise to: heart disease, bronchitis, gallstones, varicose veins and diseased joints. They are at greater risk in surgery and in childbirth and have a higher accident rate.

How do you know if you are too fat? Tables 19-21 show the acceptable range of weights for a given height, the middle weight in each range being the one recommended for good health. Anyone exceeding the upper limit is considered overweight, and obesity is defined as 20 percent more than the upper limit.

Some weight tables and weighing machines carry "desirable" weights for people of different frame sizes. As it is difficult to assess frame size, the various authorities have dropped any mention of them from their tables and give instead an "acceptable weight range"—as here.

LOSING WEIGHT

So what can be done? Everyone knows the answer to that. If gaining weight is caused by taking in more energy than you use, then taking in less energy than you use (which is not necessarily the same as taking in less food) will cause you to lose weight.

Crash or fad diets—banana diets, grapefruit diets and so on—are not much use because as soon as you stop them you will put on weight again. The same is true of drugs, which may also have undesirable side-effects.

Fasting is certainly not to be recommended unless it is done under medical supervision. Firstly, it is dangerous because in addition to fat some of the more essential parts of the body such as the tissues themselves may be used up, causing serious damage. Secondly, the body needs nutrients all the time and by fasting you would be depriving yourself of essential proteins, vitamins and minerals. And lastly, while a short fast of a few days would certainly use up some fat, this shares the disadvantage of crash diets in that you would probably resume the eating habits that made you fat in the first place.

What about exercise? If energy in minus energy out equals energy left in the body, then you should be able to lose weight by increasing energy expenditure. In practice, though, you have to exercise an awful lot to lose 2lb (1kg) of fat. It would take a 100-mile walk.

Suppose you decide to walk a fast mile or so every night after dinner instead of slumping in front of the television set. You would lose only about one-fifteenth of an ounce (2g) of weight. And if you stop at the bar on the way back don't have more than half a pint of beer, otherwise you will gain weight. If should also be remembered that exercise might give you a greater appetite.

(cont'd on page 60)

19 Desirable weights for adults*

MEN

Height		Weights in lb		
ft in	lower	average	upper	obese
5 2	112	123	141	**169**
5 3	115	127	144	**173**
5 4	118	130	148	**178**
5 5	121	133	152	**182**
5 6	124	136	156	**187**
5 7	128	140	161	**193**
5 8	132	145	166	**199**
5 9	136	149	170	**204**
5 10	140	153	174	**209**
5 11	144	158	179	**215**
6 0	148	162	184	**221**
6 1	152	166	189	**227**
6 2	156	171	194	**233**
6 3	160	176	199	**239**
6 4	164	181	204	**245**

Height m		Weights in kg		
1.58	51	55.8	64	**77**
1.60	52	57.6	65	**78**
1.62	53	58.6	66	**79**
1.64	54	59.6	67	**80**
1.66	55	60.6	69	**83**
1.68	56	61.7	71	**85**
1.70	58	63.5	73	**88**
1.72	59	65.0	74	**89**
1.74	60	66.5	75	**90**
1.76	62	68.0	77	**92**
1.78	64	69.4	79	**95**
1.80	65	71.0	80	**96**
1.82	66	72.6	82	**98**
1·84	67	74.2	84	**101**
1.86	69	75.8	86	**103**
1.88	71	77.6	88	**106**
1.90	73	79.3	90	**108**
1.92	75	81.0	93	**112**

Weights given without clothes. For indoor clothing, add: men 7-9lb (3-4kg), women 4-6lb (2.25kg). Lower and upper weights are acceptable limits for each height.

WOMEN

Height	Weights in lb			
ft in	lower	average	upper	obese
4 10	92	102	119	143
4 11	94	104	122	146
5 0	96	107	125	150
5 1	99	110	128	154
5 2	102	113	131	157
5 3	105	116	134	161
5 4	108	120	138	166
5 5	111	123	142	170
5 6	114	128	146	175
5 7	118	132	150	180
5 8	122	136	154	185
5 9	126	140	158	190
5 10	130	144	163	196
5 11	134	148	168	202
6 0	138	152	173	208

Height m	Weights in kg			
1.45	42	46.0	53	64
1.48	42	46.5	54	65
1.50	43	47.0	55	66
1.52	44	48.5	57	68
1.54	44	49.5	58	70
1.56	45	50.4	58	70
1.58	46	51.3	59	71
1.60	48	52.6	61	73
1.62	49	54.0	62	74
1.64	50	55.4	64	77
1.66	51	56.8	65	78
1.68	52	58.1	66	79
1.70	53	60.0	67	80
1.72	55	61.3	69	83
1.74	56	62.6	70	84
1.76	58	64.0	72	86
1.78	59	65.3	74	89

20 Height/weight/age table for boys of school age

Age	Heights in inches			Weights in lb		
	lower	average	upper	lower	average	upper
6	42	45	48	37	45	53
7	45	47	50	42	50	60
8	47	50	53	47	55	67
9	49	52	55	51	60	73
10	51	54	57	55	65	82
11	53	56	59	62	73	90
12	55	58	61	68	82	102
13	57	60	63	71	90	112
14	60	63	67	88	108	133
15	63	66	70	105	126	152
16	65	68	71	112	133	160
17	65	69	72	118	137	165

21 Height/weight/age table for girls of school age

Age	Heights in inches			Weights in lb		
	lower	average	upper	lower	average	upper
6	42	44	47	37	44	53
7	44	47	50	42	50	60
8	46	49	52	44	53	64
9	48	51	54	46	56	68
10	50	53	56	53	64	79
11	52	55	58	62	73	90
12	55	58	61	68	84	105
13	57	60	64	75	93	117
14	60	62	66	88	108	132
15	61	65	68	100	123	148
16	61	65	68	108	128	154
17	61	65	68	110	130	157

Age	Heights in cm			Weights in kg		
	lower	average	upper	lower	average	upper
6	108	115	122	17	20	24
7	113	120	128	19	22	27
8	119	127	134	21	25	30
9	124	132	139	23	27	33
10	129	137	145	25	30	37
11	134	142	150	28	33	41
12	139	147	155	30	37	46
13	144	152	160	32	40	51
14	152	161	170	40	49	60
15	160	169	178	47	57	68
16	164	173	181	51	60	72
17	166	175	183	53	62	74

Age	Heights in cm			Weights in kg		
	lower	average	upper	lower	average	upper
6	106	113	120	17	20	24
7	112	119	127	19	22	27
8	117	125	132	20	24	29
9	122	130	137	21	26	31
10	127	135	143	24	29	36
11	132	140	148	28	33	41
12	140	148	156	31	38	47
13	146	154	162	34	42	53
14	150	158	167	40	49	60
15	155	164	173	46	56	67
16	155	164	173	49	58	70
17	155	164	173	50	59	71

Although it is not an efficient way of losing weight, however, exercise is a useful way of preventing a weight gain. A slice of bread and butter supplies enough energy for a brisk 10-minute walk. So if our fat office worker who gained 200lb (90kg) by eating one extra slice of bread and butter a day for 20 years had also walked an extra ten minutes a day he would not have gained weight at all. (This, of course, assumes that the body behaves like an accurate weighing machine, which it doesn't, but it is a rather good illustration of the value of exercise with regard to body fat.) Of course, exercise is essential for good health, and jogging seems to be beneficial in warding off heart problems even though it does not get rid of much fat.

But if you want to lose weight, and keep it off, the only real answer is to learn to eat sensibly, and to keep these new eating habits for life.

HOW MUCH FOOD?

How much should you eat on a reducing diet? The important thing is to ensure that you are getting all the proteins, vitamins and minerals that you need without getting also too much energy. If, for instance, you normally ate about 2,500 Calories (10 megajoules) per day and reduced this to 1,250 Calories (5 megajoules), you would also be halving your usual supply of proteins, vitamins and minerals; you would have to be very careful therefore in your choice of food to ensure you were getting an adequate supply of these nutrients.

Reducing diets are usually based on about 1,200-1,500 Calories (6 megajoules) per day. With this amount it is not difficult to select foods that are rich in nutrients and low in energy value: meat, poultry, fish, cottage cheese, plenty of fruit and vegetables.

Remember that it took a long time to gain weight, so don't expect to lose it all in a few weeks. The fat office worker took 20 years to gain 200lb (90kg); a less extreme case might take a year to gain about 22lb (10kg). Even if you ate nothing at all you would lose only 12oz (0.34kg) of weight a day.

If you were about 1,000 Calories (4 megajoules) short every day you could expect to lose about 1-2lb (0.5-1kg) every week (plus some water in the first week which would make the bathroom scales look rather encouraging). Weight does not always fall steadily, but don't be discouraged—stick to it.

The main requirement for dieting is incentive and willpower. Do you really want to lose weight? No one can do it for you. If you find it difficult to reduce on your own you could join a dieter's club, such as Weight Watchers, where you learn to eat sensibly. If you really must nibble between meals, try a nibble bowl of celery, cucumber, and radishes or green peppers.

WHAT IS BROWN FAT?

Some people can eat as much as they like and never gain weight. They seem to burn off any excess food as waste heat, but we are not certain how they do it.

There is a certain amount of "brown fat" in the body—ordinary fat is nearly white—which metabolizes faster than ordinary fat and produces more heat. It seems possible, although it remains to be proved, that people who do not gain weight have more brown fat than others. In any case, whatever the reason, there is nothing one can do about it, for anyone who is overweight has no alternative but to reduce their intake of calories.

DOES DIETARY FIBER HELP?

It has been suggested that fiber-rich foods are a help in dieting, but this has never been tested. People have lost weight on a low-calorie diet rich in fiber but have not been tested on a low-calorie diet without any extra fiber.

Such a diet is worth trying, however, because fiber, in theory at least, might be helpful. It is possible that you might eat less because fiber-rich foods (such as wholegrain bread as against white bread) take longer to chew, causing more saliva to be produced; the volume reaching the stomach is greater and you might therefore feel full on less food. Finally, fiber slows down the emptying of the stomach, and as a result you might not feel hungry so soon.

Theory aside, a useful way of eating the usual amount of food while reducing your calorie intake is to eat several helpings of fruits and vegetables every day. These are bulky, low-calorie foods which will supply minerals and vitamins while helping you to feel full.

CHILDREN AND WEIGHT

Because children are growing it is necessary to take both age and height into consideration when assessing their weight. Tables 20 and 21 (pages 58–59) are collected from a number of different sources which provide the range of heights and weights considered to be acceptable for each age. They can be used only as an approximate guide. As with the table for adults (Table 19), weights in excess of 10 percent and 20 percent above the upper limit are considered to be overweight and obese respectively.

Questions
and answers

GENERAL HEALTH

Q My child won't drink milk. Will he get enough calcium from other foods?

A You get the same amount of calcium, about 250mg, which is nearly one third a child's RDA, from a glass of milk, 1oz (30g) of cheddar cheese (cream cheese and curd cheese do not contain much calcium), a 5oz (140g) carton of yogurt, or 7 slices of enriched white bread. So if these are the "other foods," yes, he can get enough.

Q My nails are soft and split easily. Will eating gelatin help strengthen them?

A There is one report of what on paper seems to have been a well-conducted trial which shows that $\frac{1}{2}$oz (15g) of gelatin a day did help to strengthen fingernails. This has neither been confirmed nor disproved, so it is worth trying.

Q I have bad acne. Are there foods I should avoid?

A We don't really know—sugary foods may be a contributory cause and so should be avoided.

Q Is it true that sufferers from migraine should not eat cheese and chocolate?

A Many foods have been shown to be a cause of migraine in different people. While chocolate, cheese and red wine have often been blamed in the past, recent trials show that almost any food can cause the problem. Sufferers should note what they have been eating just before the pain comes on, and try to work out for themselves what foods to avoid.

Q Is it true that you should "starve a fever, feed a cold?"

A No. In fact, when you are running a fever you are burning off energy at double the normal rate, so you should actually feed a fever—even though you probably don't feel much like eating.

Q Should I take extra salt or salt tablets in a hot climate?

A If you are sweating profusely, yes. Water intake is also a major problem, although your own thirst usually makes you drink. But during the first few days in such a climate your thirst may be a bit late in telling you when to drink and the sweat loss may make you feel slightly sick and unable to eat. You should therefore drink a lot of fluid, any kind, whenever sweat losses are unusually large.

Q Do you need a special diet after certain illnesses—for example, after a heart attack?

A After any illness it is essential to restore the body's reserve of nutrients, so a nutrient-rich diet is necessary for several weeks. This can be achieved by cutting down our sugar and fats and replacing them with more complete, nourishing foods.

After a heart attack it is necessary to ensure that you are not at all overweight and to restrict fatty foods severely. To be on the safe side, cholesterol intake should be limited by keeping the number of eggs per week down to four or less. Cut down also on red meat; poultry has less cholesterol.

Q Can depression be helped by a change in diet?

A This is still the subject of research and no answer is available.

Q Can a mother pass on her eating habits to her baby during pregnancy?

A No, not so far as we know.

Q Should I change my eating habits during pregnancy?

A Depends on how bad they were before. You need a "balanced diet"—see below.

Q Is it true that nothing in itself is bad for you, but that some things are better for you than others?

A In small amounts nothing is bad for you, even alcohol. It is when you take abnormally large amounts of particular foods that they may themselves cause harm. They push the better foods out of the diet.

Q Does a large dose of vitamin C prevent a cold?

A Unfortunately, no. A few experiments suggest that doses of 1g or so of vitamin C might shorten a cold or lessen the symptoms, but there is no clear evidence.

NUTRITION

Q What is meant by a balanced diet?

A Simply a good diet, with enough of all the nutrients—protein, vitamins and mineral salts—rather than one overloaded with fat or carbohydrate and relatively short of many of these nutrients.

Q Is an irregular diet necessarily a bad thing?

A In theory the body should receive a regular supply of nutrients—three meals a day—but many people manage very well indeed on one meal a day or even when eating irregularly. Probably it would be better if they did eat regularly.

Q Is it true that if you are going to eat one big meal a day

it ought to be breakfast so that you have time to burn it up during the day?
A It does not matter and is largely a matter of habit.

Q Is it true that you should not eat and drink together, that is, is it better to drink before (or after) a meal?
A It does not matter.

Q How much protein is good for you? Is it possible to eat too much protein?
A The amount of protein that we need is only about 6-7 percent of the diet, but that would not be very palatable. On average we consume about 12-15 percent of our food in the form of protein. Taking more, however, is neither good nor bad.

Q Why do some foods upset certain people?
A Some people are allergic to certain foods, either natural or processed, or to some food additives (such as the yellow colour, tartrazine, which can affect perhaps one person in every few thousand). Most other people are quite un-affected by these, so for the vast majority of people the additives are quite safe—and one could hardly ban meat, milk or tea, or whatever foods affect some people. They should find out which foods or which additives affect them and refrain from consuming them.

Q Is a varied diet better than a stable one? Wild animals, after all, live well on the same food all the time.
A In order to get all the nutrients we need we have to consume a large number of different foods, for no single food supplies all the necessary nutrients. People on mono-tonous diets sometimes suffer from nutritional defici-encies. Farm animals and our pets are usually fed a complete mixture containing all the required nutrients, especially nowadays when we know fairly exactly what nutrients they need. But even if we knew exactly what is required for our own good health we would hardly enjoy eating a packet of complete nutrients at every meal.

Q Is butter better than margarine?
A On the contrary, margarine is richer in vitamin D than butter because it is added by law; it is as rich as summer butter in vitamin A, and thus richer than winter butter; and special margarines are rich in polyunsaturated fatty acids, while butter is far more saturated.

Q Why is brown bread considered healthier than white?
A Because it contains more of the B vitamins, iron and dietary fiber. Enriched white bread is not as rich in these as whole-grain bread. Some brown breads are not much better than white, and others are close to whole-grain; the word "brown" covers a range of breads.

Q Why is brown rice better than white rice?
A White rice is made by milling the bran from brown rice, the rice germ being lost at the same time. This reduces the amount of B vitamins and fiber. Some specially prepared products fall in between, and in some countries white rice is enriched with B vitamins.

Q Is brown sugar better for you than white sugar?
A There is no measurable difference. Both are nearly 100-percent sucrose.

DIETING

Q How fat can you get?
A One of the fattest men ever was William Campbell of Britain who reached 750 lb or 340 kg in 1878.

This enormous weight gave him about 2 million Calories of surplus fat, but because he died at the age of 22 he could have built up this store by eating only 250 surplus Calories each day of his life.

Q Is it helpful to take weight-reducing drugs?
A For most people, no. There is a strong risk of side effects, and when they stop taking the drug they tend to return to the wrong eating habits that made them fat in the first place.

Q Will I lose weight if I exercise regularly?
A Usually, yes, but not much. See the section on losing weight in OBESITY AND DIETING.

Q Would skipping a meal help me to lose weight?
A No. Skipping meals usually results in eating more at the next meal—or between meals. Better to learn improved eating habits at all meals.

Q Will it help me to lose weight if I eat more slowly?
A No, but what it might do is make you eat less. If you overeat because you love food, slowly savoring each mouthful might lead to a smaller intake. But if you are fat because your needs are small then it will probably have no effect at all.

Q When dieting, should you avoid salt because it leads to water retention?
A In a healthy person, even if obese, water and salt balance themselves automatically, and the body contains a fairly constant amount of water. Extra salt simply causes more thirst and both are excreted. But generally we all eat too much salt.

Q Does constipation make you fat?
A No: it might cause a bulge but it does not make any fatty tissue.

Q Will I put on weight if I give up smoking?

A Many people put on weight when they stop smoking. For some people this is because they eat more, because smoking depresses the appetite and tends to spoil the taste of food. But even if you do not eat any more you may still gain weight because smoking has some effect in speeding up the metabolism and burning up food a little faster.

Q How can you measure your metabolism, and can it be altered?

A Metabolism can easily be measured in the laboratory or hospital, but unfortunately it cannot be altered. Some people are unluckily born with a slow metabolic rate, so they need only, say, 1,500 Calories a day compared to the average of about 2,300. They would actually gain weight on the average diet, and even on an ordinary reducing diet. Others are born with the ability to burn off any extra food they eat.

Q Are there any special dieting foods? Is it true that a grapefruit before a meal will burn up the carbohydrate?

A No food is reducing. Some foods supply less energy than others, so it does help to replace energy-dense foods that contain sugar or fats with low-energy foods, such as vegetables and many fruits.

There is nothing in the idea of the grapefruit diet—or the potato diet, pineapple diet or any other similar fad.

Recipes for better health

Recipe books are usually intended to improve cooking skills and add to the variety of the diet. Here we provide a selection of recipes that should achieve both these objectives while at the same time improving the diet nutritionally.

> Some of the recipes are:
> low in fat—marked ●
> low in salt—marked ▲
> low in sugar—marked ■

Very often a reduction in fat and sugar will automatically reduce calorie-intake, because these two ingredients are concentrated energy.

It is easy to plan an attractive, palatable diet that fulfills the desired nutritional goals (see pages 22-23). It is a matter of selecting the right foods while reducing the amount of wrong foods, and using recipes that point in this direction. Weight reduction and "healthy eating" need be neither painful nor unappetizing.

Low-fat spreads, low-fat cheese and low-fat milk (which is 2-percent fat, instead of 4-percent as in full-cream milk) as well as skimmed milk are widely available, and can help to reduce energy and fat intake. While it is true that low-fat spreads are simply ordinary margarine-type fats with added water and air so that they collapse when heated, they are useful for sautéing because the water in the spread helps to cover the food.

Many standard recipes can be improved nutritionally by simply reducing the amounts of sugar and fat, and proportionately increasing the other ingredients. Similarly the salt can often be reduced: salting food is largely a matter of habit.

Hors d'oeuvre

CHICKEN-LIVER PÂTÉ

4oz (110g) chicken livers
2oz (60g) onion, chopped
1 egg, hard-boiled
Pinch of salt; pepper to taste
1 teaspoon low-fat spread

Place the livers and onion in a saucepan with one tablespoon of water. Cook gently until tender. Drain well, add salt and pepper, and mince together with the egg. Add the low-fat spread, mash well with a fork and serve cold on a bed of lettuce.

Calories per serving: 130   **Serves 2**

MACKEREL PÂTÉ

4oz (110g) smoked mackerel filets
½ garlic clove, crushed
Black pepper to taste
2 teaspoons lemon juice
1oz (30g) low-fat yogurt

Skin filets, chop roughly, add other ingredients and pound well until soft.

Calories per serving: 120   **Serves 2**

"FRENCH" MUSHROOMS ● ▲

4oz (110g) button mushrooms
1oz (30g) low-fat spread
1 garlic clove, crushed
Dash of black pepper

Place all the ingredients in a small pan, bring to the boil, stirring well, cover and cook gently until tender (about 6 minutes). Serve at once.

Calories per serving: 120   **Serves 2**

SHRIMP IN TOMATOES

4 large tomatoes
4oz (110g) peeled cooked shrimp
2 tablespoons low-calorie salad dressing
4 tablespoons canned sweetcorn
Salt and pepper
Lettuce leaves, finely shredded

Cut the tops off the tomatoes and set them aside. Using a metal teaspoon, scoop the insides out of the tomatoes, being careful to keep the shells intact. Discard the insides. Mix the shrimp, salad dressing, corn, salt and pepper together and pile the mixture into the tomato shells. Replace the tomato tops. Arrange on shredded lettuce. Serve chilled.

Calories per serving: 130   **Serves 2**

SHRIMP SURPRISE ●

8 large Pacific shrimp, cooked and peeled
8 lettuce leaves
¼ garlic clove, crushed
2 tablespoons white wine vinegar

Red and yellow peppers (capsicum), thinly sliced

Mix the vinegar and garlic together. Roll each shrimp in a lettuce leaf, place 4 on each plate, garnish with the sliced peppers and pour the garlic vinegar over them.

Calories per serving: 70   **Serves 2**

MOULES MARINIÈRES ●

12 fl. oz (340 ml) dry white wine
4 fl. oz (110 ml) water
2 garlic cloves, crushed
2 tablespoons chopped fresh parsley
2 bay leaves
4 tomatoes, chopped
Pepper
24 large mussels

Put all the ingredients except the mussels in a shallow pan. Cover the pan and bring the liquid to the boil. Reduce the heat and simmer for 5 minutes. Meanwhile, scrub the mussels clean and tug out the "beards." Give them a final rinse in a large bowl of cold water and drain well. Remove the pan from the heat and pour the liquid through a strainer. Discard the contents of the strainer and return the liquid to the shallow pan. Arrange the mussels in the pan and cover. Steam over moderate heat for about 6 minutes until they open. Discard any mussels which have not opened. Serve immediately.

Calories per serving: 260   **Serves 2**

For more hors d'oeuvre ideas, see the section on Salads.

Soups

WATERCRESS AND YOGURT SOUP ● ▲

2 large bunches watercress, chopped
½ pint (3 dl) water
½ pint (3 dl) low-fat natural yogurt
Pepper

Put the watercress and water into a saucepan and simmer for 15 minutes. Blend the contents in a blender, or rub them through a strainer, and return to the pan. Stir in the yogurt, add pepper to taste, reheat over low heat and serve.

Calories per serving: 75   **Serves 2**

CONSOMMÉ WITH VEGETABLES ●

1 can consommé (beef or chicken)

> 2 medium carrots, diced
> 1 medium leek, finely chopped
> 2 tomatoes, chopped
> Salt and pepper

Put all the ingredients except the salt and pepper into a saucepan and simmer, covered, over low heat until the vegetables are tender but not mushy. Taste the soup and if necessary add salt and pepper. Serve hot.

Calories per serving: 60   **Serves 2**

LEEK AND TOMATO SOUP ● ▲

> 2 large leeks, finely chopped
> 2 large tomatoes, chopped
> 1 bay leaf
> Pinch of dried mixed herbs
> 5fl.oz (140ml) water
> 5fl.oz (140ml) low-fat natural yogurt
> Pepper

Put the vegetables, herbs and water into a saucepan and simmer, covered, until the vegetables are tender. Discard the bay leaf and blend the mixture in a blender, or rub it through a strainer. Return the soup to the pan, and stir in the yogurt and pepper to taste. Reheat over low heat and serve.

Calories per serving: 50   **Serves 2**

CELERY SOUP ●

> 15oz (450g) can of celery, well drained
> 1 pint (½ liter) low-fat milk
> Salt and pepper to taste
> Large sprig of parsley

Blend celery and milk, season to taste, heat gently to boiling point and serve sprinkled with parsley.

Calories per serving: 100   **Serves 2**

Egg and cheese dishes

BASIC OMELET

> 4 small eggs
> Pepper
> 2 tablespoons water
> ½oz (15g) butter

Beat the eggs, pepper and water together. Heat the butter over moderate heat in an omelet pan, swirling it around so that it coats the bottom of the pan. Pour in the beaten eggs and stir lightly with a fork for the first few seconds. When the bottom of the omelet is beginning to set, lift up one edge with a spatula and tip the runny egg in that direction. Put the pan straight over the flame again and, if you like, sprinkle with a filling (see below). When the omelet is cooked, flip it over quickly with a spatula so that it is folded in half. Serve immediately on a hot plate.

Calories per serving: 200   **Serves 2**

OMELET FILLINGS

Even with the fillings the omelets are still low in calories.

Chicken
4oz (110g) diced cooked chicken
4 scallions, finely shredded
Calories per serving: 290   **Serves 2**

Fines herbes
2 teaspoons each fresh chopped
parsley, thyme and tarragon
Calories per serving: 200   **Serves 2**

Cheese and tomato
2 large tomatoes, finely chopped
2oz (60g) low-fat cheese, grated
Calories per serving: 290   **Serves 2**

Mushroom
4oz (110g) button mushrooms, halved,
poached and drained
1 shallot, very finely sliced
Calories per serving: 210   **Serves 2**

Beef and asparagus
4oz (110g) lean beef, diced
4 sticks asparagus, fresh and chopped,
or canned without added salt
Calories per serving: 250   **Serves 2**

Shrimp
4oz (110g) peeled cooked shrimp
4 teaspoons chopped fresh chives
Calories per serving: 260   **Serves 2**

SPANISH OMELET

3 tablespoons butter
2 shallots (or 1 small onion), finely chopped
1 canned pimiento, chopped
4oz (110g) cooked green beans, chopped
4oz (110g) button mushrooms, halved
Pepper
4 eggs

Melt 2 tablespoons of the butter in a saucepan, and add the vegetables and pepper. Fry gently until the vegetables are cooked. Remove the pan from the heat. Melt the remaining butter in an omelet pan. Beat the eggs and a little pepper together with a fork and pour them into the omelet pan. Stir the eggs lightly with a fork until the bottom of the omelet is just beginning to set. Sprinkle the vegetables over the top of the omelet and serve when the egg has set.

Calories per serving: 360   **Serves 2**

LEMON SOUFFLÉ OMELET

4 eggs, separated
Juice and finely grated rind of 2 large lemons
Liquid sweetener to taste
1 tablespoon butter

Put the egg yolks, lemon juice and rind, and sweetener in a bowl. Beat well with a fork, then beat the egg whites until stiff, and using a metal spoon, fold in. Melt the butter in an omelet pan and pour in the mixture. Cook over low heat until the bottom has set and looks lightly browned. Remove the pan from the heat and hold it under a moderately hot grill until the top is browned and set. The middle should be slightly runny. Serve immediately.

Calories per serving: 210   **Serves 3**

SCRAMBLED EGGS WITH ASPARAGUS

4 eggs
Pepper
½ teaspoon paprika
2 tablespoons water
12 large asparagus spears, steamed
½oz (15g) butter, melted

Beat the eggs, salt, pepper, paprika and water together with a fork. Scramble over moderate heat in a saucepan. Put the scrambled egg on a warmed plate. Lay the asparagus spears down beside the egg, pour the melted butter over and serve.

Calories per serving: 230   **Serves 2**

HUEVOS FLAMENCOS ▲

4 eggs
1oz (30g) fresh or frozen peas
1oz (30g) frozen or canned (unsweetened) sweetcorn
1oz (30g) precooked or frozen carrots, diced
Black pepper to taste
Small quantity of low-fat spread

Take 2 fairly shallow ovenproof dishes, large enough to

allow the eggs to spread out, and grease the dishes sparsely with the low-fat spread. Break 2 eggs into each dish, keeping the yolks whole. Sprinkle half the vegetables onto each dish and shake on a little pepper. Bake in a moderate oven (350°F/180°C) until the whites are hard and the yolks just set. Serve hot.

Calories per serving: 170   **Serves 2**

SCRAMBLED EGGS WITH SMOKED SALMON

4 eggs
1 tablespoon chopped fresh chives
2 tablespoons milk
4oz (110g) smoked salmon, cut into thin strips

Beat the eggs, chives and milk together and put them in a saucepan. Scramble over low heat. When the eggs are nearly scrambled, stir in the smoked salmon. Serve hot.

Calories per serving: 260   **Serves 2**

MACARONI CHEESE ●▲

4oz (110g) macaroni
¾ pint (4dl) skimmed milk
¾oz (20g) margarine
1oz (30g) plain flour
4oz (110g) low-fat cheese

Boil the macaroni and drain off the water. Make white sauce from the milk, flour and margarine (see Basic sauces, page 80). Add ¾ of the cheese, then the macaroni, sprinkle the rest of the cheese on top and brown under the grill.

Calories per serving: 150   **Serves 3**

CAULIFLOWER CHEESE ●▲

½ small cauliflower (about 12oz/340g)
¼ pint (140ml) skimmed milk
½oz (10g) margarine
½oz (15g) plain flour
2oz (60g) low-fat cheese, grated
Pinch of pepper

Boil the cauliflower until tender, drain, retaining about 1½ fl. oz (50ml) of the water, and keep the cauliflower hot. Make a white sauce from the flour, margarine, and cauliflower water topped up with the milk (see Basic sauces, page 80). Add ¾ of the cheese, with pepper to season, and pour over the cauliflower. Sprinkle the remaining grated cheese over the top, and brown under the grill.

Calories per serving: 160   **Serves 2**

Meat, poultry and fish dishes

DIETER'S HAMBURGER (1) ●▲

8oz (230g) lean ground beef
1 small onion, very finely chopped
2 teaspoons water
Freshly ground black pepper

Preheat the grill to moderate. Mix all the ingredients well with your hands and shape into two balls. Flatten the balls between the palms of your hands and place on the grill rack. Grill for about 3 minutes on each side, or more, depending on how well done you like your meat. Season to taste. Serve hot or cold.

Calories per serving: 150   **Serves 2**

DIETER'S HAMBURGER (2)

8oz (230g) lean ground beef
1 medium egg
1oz (30g) onion, chopped
1 teaspoon mixed dried herbs
½ slice whole-grain bread, crumbed
Salt and pepper to taste

Place the meat, onion, herbs, salt and pepper in a bowl. Make a hole in the middle, break in the egg and mix well together. Shape the meat mixture into 2 balls and flatten them between the palms of your hands. Grill to taste, depending on how well done you like your meat.

Calories per serving: 180   **Serves 2**

BEEF AND VEGETABLE STEW ●▲

8oz (230g) lean beef, cut into small cubes
2 large tomatoes, chopped
2 leeks, finely chopped
4oz (110g) button mushrooms
4fl.oz (110ml) water
Pepper
2 small bay leaves

Place the onion, peppers and mushrooms on the veal over low heat for about 25 minutes, or until the beef is cooked and some of the liquid has evaporated to make the stew thicker.

Calories per serving: 160   **Serves 2**

BEEF GOULASH ●▲

8oz (230g) lean beef, cut into small cubes
2 small bay leaves

Pepper
2 tablespoons paprika
½ pint (3dl) low-fat natural yogurt
2 medium-sized potatoes, peeled and cut into small cubes
2 small onions, very thinly sliced

Put all the ingredients into a saucepan and mix well. Simmer over low heat, uncovered, for about 25 minutes, or until the beef and potatoes are cooked and the stew has thickened.

Calories per serving: 300 **Serves 2**

SPICED BEEF

8oz (230g) filet steak, thinly sliced and cut into strips
2 tablespoons soy sauce
2 tablespoons lemon juice
3 tablespoons olive oil
1 green pepper, finely chopped
1 tablespoon finely chopped fresh ginger root
1 large garlic clove, chopped
8oz (230g) bean sprouts, steamed

Put the steak in a small, shallow dish and pour the soy sauce and lemon juice over it. Stir well to mix, and marinate, stirring occasionally, for 1 hour. Drain the meat and set it aside. Heat the oil in a small frying-pan and add the pepper, ginger and garlic. Fry, stirring constantly, for 2 minutes. Add the beef and continue frying until it is cooked. Put the bean sprouts on a plate and add the meat. Serve hot.

Calories per serving: 350 **Serve 2**

VEAL PIMIENTOS ● ▲

2 thin 4oz (110g) slices of veal
2oz (60g) onion, chopped
6oz (170g) green peppers, chopped
4oz (110g) button (or larger sliced) mushrooms
2½oz (75g) tomato purée, mixed with ½ pint (3dl) water
1 teaspoon mixed Italian seasoning; black pepper to taste

Place the onion, peppers and mushrooms on the veal slices and roll into sausage shapes. Place in a baking dish and cover with the diluted, seasoned purée. Bake at 425°F/220°C for about 40 minutes or until tender.

Calories per serving: 170 **Serves 2**

VEAL AND MUSHROOMS ● ▲

12oz (340g) veal filet, cut into strips
4 small shallots, very finely sliced
4oz (110g) button mushrooms, halved

½ pint (3dl) low-fat natural yogurt
2 teaspoons paprika

Preheat the oven to 375°F/190°C. Mix all the ingredients except the paprika together and put them into a baking dish. Sprinkle over the paprika. Cover the dish with foil and bake for 25 minutes, or until the veal is tender. Serve hot.

Calories per serving: 270   **Serves 2**

CHICKEN CURRY ● ▲

6oz (170g) cooked chicken, diced (without skin)
4 tomatoes, chopped
4oz (110g) button mushrooms, halved
2 garlic cloves, crushed
1 teaspoon ground cumin
2 teaspoons garam masala
½ teaspoon chili powder
2 tablespoons water
4fl.oz (110ml) low-fat natural yogurt
8oz (230g) boiled bean sprouts, hot (or canned and heated)

Mix all the ingredients except the bean sprouts together in a saucepan. Cover the pan and simmer for 20 minutes, stirring occasonally. Put the bean sprouts on a warmed plate and pour over the curry. Serve immediately.

Calories per serving: 200   **Serves 2**

SPICED GRILLED CHICKEN ●

1 tablespoon soy sauce
2 teaspoons lemon juice
2 teaspoons prepared mustard
1 garlic clove, crushed
2 small chicken breasts (about 4oz/110g each)

Mix the soy sauce, lemon juice, mustard and garlic to a paste and spread them all over the chicken. Set aside in a cool place for 1 hour (this will allow the flavorings to seep into the meat). Preheat the grill to moderate. Line the grill rack with foil and place the chicken on it. Grill for about 7 minutes on each side, or until the chicken is cooked. Serve hot or cold.

Calories per serving: 200   **Serves 2**

STUFFED EGGPLANT OR SQUASH ● ▲

2 eggplants or small squash (3-4oz/90-110g)
8oz (230g) cold meat or chicken, chopped
1oz (30g) onion, chopped
1 garlic clove, crushed
2oz (60g) low-fat cheese, grated

1 tablespoon tomato purée

Cook eggplants or squash gently until tender enough to scoop out without damaging skin. Cut in half and scoop out. Mix with all other ingredients except cheese and pile back in. Sprinkle with cheese and bake at 400°F/200°C for 25 minutes or until golden brown.
Calories per serving: 300   **Serves 2**

"TARRAGON WINE" LIVER ▲

12oz (340g) calf liver, thinly sliced
2oz (60g) onion, chopped
1 dessertspoon (10ml) red wine vinegar
Large sprig of parsley, chopped
1 teaspoon tarragon, chopped or dried
1oz (30g) low-fat spread
Black pepper to taste

Melt the low-fat spread in a medium saucepan. Add the onion and cook gently until tender. Add the liver and sauté for about 5 minutes. Then add the vinegar and tarragon, season with pepper and cook for a further 2 minutes. Serve hot, sprinkled with parsley.
Calories per serving: 370   **Serves 2**

COD IN PARSLEY SAUCE ● ▲

12oz (340g) cod steak
8oz (230g) boiled new potatoes, hot
½ pint (3dl) low-calorie white sauce, hot
(see Basic sauces, page 80)
2 tablespoons freshly chopped parsley

Poach the cod lightly in a little water. Drain and put on a heated plate. Surround with the potatoes. Mix the sauce with the parsley, pour over the fish and serve immediately.
Calories per serving: 290   **Serves 2**

COD ALMONDESA ▲

12oz (6oz/170g each) cod (or haddock) filets
2 tablespoons parsley, chopped
2oz (60g) low-fat spread
2 tablespoons lemon juice
1oz (30g) almond flakes
½ fresh lemon

Place the fish in an ovenproof dish, pour the lemon juice over, dab the fat over the fish, and sprinkle with parsley and almond flakes. Bake at 400°F/200°C for about 25 minutes. Serve with a ¼ lemon wedge on the side.
Calories per serving: 320   **Serves 2**

Salads

CHICKEN SALAD ● ▲

4fl.oz (110ml) low-fat natural yogurt
2 teaspoons lemon juice
Pepper
8oz (230g) cooked chicken, cut into strips
2 bunches mustard greens

Mix the yogurt, lemon juice and pepper together. Put all the remaining ingredients in a bowl, pour the yogurt dressing over, toss well and serve.

Calories per serving: 230   **Serves 2**

CURRIED CHICKEN MAYONNAISE ● ▲

3 tablespoons low-calorie mayonnaise
1 tablespoon lemon juice
1 tablespoon curry powder
12oz (340g) cooked chicken meat, cut into strips
4 large lettuce leaves
4 medium tomatoes, sliced

Mix the mayonnaise, lemon juice and curry powder together in a bowl. Add the chicken and stir well to mix. Line a plate with the lettuce leaves and pile the chicken mixture in the middle. Arrange the sliced tomatoes around the edge of the plate and serve.

Calories per serving: 240   **Serves 2**

SALMON SALAD ▲

4 large lettuce leaves
12oz (340g) salmon steak, poached in a little water
with 1 tablespoon vinegar or lemon juice
8 large radishes, sliced
4 tomatoes, sliced
8 scallions
1 lemon, cut into wedges

Lay the lettuce leaves on a plate and put the salmon steak on top. Arrange the salad vegetables and lemon wedges decoratively around the salmon, and serve.

Calories per serving: 360   **Serves 2**

COLESLAW SALAD ● ▲

2 tablespoons low-calorie salad dressing
¼ teaspoon prepared mustard
Pepper
4oz (110g) white cabbage, coarsely shredded
2 medium carrots, shredded

1 small onion, very thinly sliced

Mix the salad dressing, mustard and pepper together and add the vegetables. Toss well, chill and serve.

Calories per serving: 50   **Serves 2**

CARROT, APPLE AND NUT SALAD ▲

12oz (340g) raw carrot, peeled and grated
1oz (30g) fresh peanuts
2 small eating apples, cored and diced
2 teaspoons lemon juice
1 tablespoon cider vinegar
Pepper

Mix all the ingredients together, chill and serve.

Calories per serving: 220   **Serves 2**

ENDIVE SALAD ▲

2 teaspoons olive oil
1 tablespoon tarragon vinegar
Pepper
½ teaspoon prepared mustard
1 small curly endive, chopped
2oz (60g) small mushrooms, thinly sliced
½oz (15g) peanuts, chopped

Mix the olive oil, vinegar, pepper and mustard together. Put all the vegetables and nuts in a salad bowl, pour over the dressing, toss well and serve.

Calories per serving: 80   **Serves 2**

ENDIVE AND WALNUT SALAD ▲

½ small curly endive, coarsely chopped
1oz (30g) chopped walnuts
2oz (60g) raw button mushrooms, thinly sliced
1 tablespoon olive oil
2 teaspoons lemon juice
1 tablespoon vinegar
2 teaspoons French mustard
1 garlic clove, crushed; pepper

Put the endive, walnuts and mushrooms into a salad bowl. Mix the remaining dressing ingredients together and pour them over the salad. Toss well and serve.

Calories per serving: 130   **Serves 2**

CHEESE, ORANGE AND WATERCRESS SALAD

4 tablespoons low-fat natural yogurt
2 tablespoons lemon juice

Pepper
2 bunches watercress, chopped
2 large oranges, peeled and chopped
4oz (110g) Edam cheese, chopped

Mix the yogurt, lemon juice, salt and pepper together in a small salad bowl. Add the remaining ingredients, toss well and serve.

Calories per serving: 200   **Serves 2**

CHICORY, ORANGE AND WATERCRESS SALAD ● ▲

2 heads chicory, thinly sliced
2 oranges, peeled, halved and thinly sliced
2 bunches watercress, chopped
1 tablespoon tarragon vinegar
2 teaspoons lemon juice
1 teaspoon French mustard
Pepper

Put the chicory, orange and watercress into a salad bowl. Mix the remaining ingredients together and pour them over the salad. Toss well and serve.

Calories per serving: 60   **Serves 2**

Basic sauces

LOW-CALORIE WHITE SAUCE

½ pint (3dl) skimmed milk
1oz (30g) all-purpose flour
½oz (15g) margarine

Melt the fat in a saucepan, add the flour and cook for a few minutes, stirring constantly. Then slowly add the milk, stirring slowly, and cook over a low heat until the sauce thickens.

Calories per fl. oz: 40

May be used to make savory sauces by adding tomato purée, meat stock, half-fat cheese, etc.

LOW-CALORIE ONION SAUCE

½ pint (3dl) skimmed milk
1oz (30g) all-purpose flour
1oz (30g) margarine
7oz (200g) onion, chopped and boiled
¼ teaspoon salt; pepper to taste

Make white sauce as above, adding the onion when the

sauce is cooked to the correct smoothness, and stir well.
Calories per fl.oz: 25

Desserts and cakes

FRUIT CREAM ●▲■

2oz (60g) dried skimmed milk
4oz (110g) fruit (strawberries, raspberries, black
currants or cooked apples), fresh or frozen
½oz (15g) gelatin
½ pint (3dl) water, warmed
Liquid sweetener to taste

Melt the gelatin in the warmed water. Mash the fruit in a
blender, add milk and sweetener, and whip the mixture
until it is creamy in texture.
Calories per fl.oz: 15   **Serves 2**

GOOSEBERRY FOOL ●▲■

1lb (450g) dessert gooseberries
2 tablespoons water
½ pint (3dl) low-fat natural yogurt
Liquid sweetener to taste

Put the gooseberries and water into a saucepan and cover
the pan. Cook over low heat until the gooseberries are
quite mushy. Remove the pan from the heat and mash the
gooseberries with a fork until they form a purée. Stir in the
yogurt and enough sweetener to taste. Chill before
serving.
Calories per serving: 160   **Serves 2**

PLUM COMPOTE ●▲■

1lb (450g) ripe dessert plums, halved and pitted
Grated rind of 1 lemon
Pinch of allspice
4 tablespoons water

Put all the ingredients in a saucepan and cover the pan.
Cook over gentle heat until the plums are very tender and
beginning to go mushy. Chill and serve.
Calories per serving: 80   **Serves 2**

APPLE AND ORANGE COMPOTE ●▲■

4 medium cooking apples, peeled, cored and sliced
2oz (60g) raisins
Juice and grated rind of 1 large orange

Liquid sweetener to taste

Put the apples, raisins, orange rind and juice into a saucepan. Cover the pan and simmer until the apples are tender and beginning to disintegrate. Remove the pan from the heat and add sweetener to taste. Serve chilled.

Calories per serving: 140   **Serves 2**

FRUIT "ICE" ●▲■

5oz (140g) low-fat natural yogurt
½oz (15g) gelatin
1 teaspoon lemon juice
4oz (110g) fruit (strawberries, raspberries, black currants or cooked apples), fresh or frozen
Liquid sweetener to taste

Melt the gelatin in 2 tablespoons warm water, and add the lemon juice and yogurt. Mash the fruit in a blender, add the sweetener, then blend in the gelatin-and-yogurt mix until the consistency is fluffy. Chill and serve.

Calories per serving: 75   **Serves 2**

ICED MELON MOUSSE ●▲■

12oz (340g) wedge of honeydew melon
1 teaspoon ground ginger
Liquid sweetener to taste
4 egg whites, stiffly whipped

Scoop the flesh out of the melon and blend it in a blender, or rub it through a strainer. Put the puréed melon into a bowl and stir in the ginger, with enough liquid sweetener to taste. Fold in the egg whites and pour the mixture into a small dish. Chill for 2 hours before serving.

Calories per serving: 50   **Serves 2**

RASPBERRY CREAM ●▲■

8oz (230g) fresh raspberries
½ pint (3dl) low-fat yogurt
Liquid sweetener to taste

Mash the raspberries with a fork and stir them into the yogurt. Add enough sweetener to taste. Serve chilled.

Calories per serving: 60

APRICOT MOUSSE ●▲■

3oz (90g) dried apricot halves
½ pint (3dl) water
4 strips lemon rind
8fl.oz (230ml) low-fat natural yogurt

2 large egg whites, stiffly whipped

Soak the apricots in the water for 2 hours. Put the apricots and water in a saucepan with the lemon rind, and simmer until the apricots are very tender and beginning to turn mushy. Rub the mixture through a strainer and let it cool. Stir in the yogurt and then fold in the egg whites. Chill before serving.

Calories per serving: 150   **Serves 2**

PRUNE WHIP ●▲■

4oz (110g) dried pitted prunes
½ pint (3dl) water
4 strips orange rind
½ pint (3dl) low-fat natural yogurt

Soak the prunes in the water for 2 hours. Put the prunes and water into a saucepan with the orange rind. Cover the pan and simmer until the prunes are very tender and beginning to go mushy. Rub them through a strainer. Using a fork, beat in the yogurt. Chill before serving.

Calories per serving: 160   **Serves 2**

APPLE SNOW ●▲■

8oz (230g) sweet eating apples, peeled and cored
Grated orange or lemon rind
2 tablespoons water
1 large egg white, stiffly beaten

Slice the apples thinly and put them in a saucepan with the rind and water. Cover the pan and cook gently, stirring occasionally, until the apples are soft. Rub the apples through a strainer and let them cool. Fold in the egg white and chill before serving.

Calories per serving: 90   **Serves 2**

EGG CUSTARD ▲■

7fl.oz (200ml) low-fat milk
2 eggs (small)
Liquid sweetener to taste
2 drops vanilla extract (optional)

Mix all the ingredients together thoroughly in a small heat-proof bowl. Set the bowl over a pan of barely simmering water and cook, stirring constantly, until the custard is thick enough to coat the back of the spoon. Pour into a small dish. Serve hot or cold.

This can be flavored with strong black coffee or cocoa powder to make coffee cream or chocolate cream.

Calories per serving: 125
Makes about 9fl.oz (260ml).   **Serves 2**

LOW-CALORIE CUSTARD ●▲■

½ pint (3dl) low-fat milk
2 drops vanilla extract
2 teaspoons cornflour, mixed with 1 tablespoon water
Liquid sweetener to taste

Put the milk, vanilla extract and cornflour into a small saucepan and cook over moderate heat, stirring, until the custard has thickened. Remove the pan from the heat and stir in sweetener to taste. Serve hot or cold.

Calories per serving: 80   **Serves 2**

SCOTCH PANCAKES

8oz (230g) self-raising flour
1 tablespoon sugar
2 eggs
Approx ⅓ pint (2dl) milk
Pinch of salt

Place dry ingredients in a bowl and add eggs. Beat, gradually adding milk, until a fairly stiff batter is achieved. Either fry in *very shallow* corn oil or cook on a griddle.

Calories each: 25   **Makes 25**

DROP SCONES ●▲■

7oz (200g) all-purpose flour
1½oz (45g) margarine
⅓ pint (200ml) skimmed milk
1 egg
½oz (15g) caster sugar
Pinch (less than ¼ teaspoon) salt
½ level teaspoon baking powder (bicarbonate of soda)
1 level teaspoon cream of tartar

Sift the flour with the baking powder and cream of tartar, rub in the fat and mix in the caster sugar. Stir in the milk and egg, and beat to a stiff batter. Drop the batter by the teaspoonful onto a hot griddle greased with not more than ½oz (15g) of margarine.

Calories each: 40   **Makes about 30 ½oz**
                                       (15g) scones

Food composition and Calorie tables

The tables in this section answer the often-asked question: Is such-and-such a good food? There is no *yes* or *no* answer because almost all foods supply *some* nutrients.

HOW TO USE THE TABLES

How much food is on the plate—or in the packet? Once you have an accurate weight or measure, use the full tables as in the abbreviated example on this page. The 12 tables are listed on the CONTENTS page at the beginning of the book.

1 To check the basic *nutritional value* of the food, look for these **1 oz (30g)** measures—or equivalent convenient small portions, e.g., **1 egg, 1 teaspoon of yeast extract,** etc. Then look along the line. ○ = **3% of Recommended Daily Allowance;** ● = **10% of RDA.** Thus 1 oz (30g) of raw beef steak provides 3% of RDA for **protein, iron** and **riboflavin,** and 10% of RDA for **niacin.**

3 Portions containing 500 Calories or more are rated as *main dishes*. Look along the line: ○ = $\frac{1}{3}$ **of RDA;** ● = $\frac{2}{3}$ **of RDA.** Thus 8 oz (230 g) of fried beef provides $\frac{1}{3}$ of RDA for **iron** and **riboflavin,** and $\frac{2}{3}$ of RDA for **protein** and **niacin.**

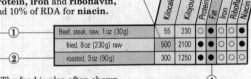

	Kilocalories	Kilojoules	Protein	Fat	Iron	Riboflavin	Niacin
(1) Beef, steak, raw, 1 oz (30g)	55	230	○	●	○	○	●
fried, 8 oz (230g) raw	500	2100	●	●	○	○	●
(2) roasted, 3 oz (90g)	300	1250	●	●	○	○	○

(3) (4)

2 The food is also often shown in *portions*. Usually these are **4 oz (110g),** but sometimes they are either more or less—as here. Now look along the line. ○ = $\frac{1}{6}$ **of RDA;** ● = $\frac{1}{2}$ **of RDA.** Thus 3 oz (90g) of roasted beef provides $\frac{1}{6}$ of RDA for **iron, riboflavin** and **niacin,** and $\frac{1}{2}$ of RDA for **protein.**

4 In the **Fat** column, ○ indicates that $\frac{1}{3}$ of the total calories for this amount of food comes from fat, ● that $\frac{2}{3}$ comes from fat. Remember that the *amount eaten* is very important.

Take note The above examples show how the values of the ○ and ● symbols vary according to whether you are looking for the basic *nutritional value* of the food, measuring the value of a *portion* or a *main dish*, or checking the *fat* content. So it is essential to measure the **weight** of the food accurately, and to be clear about the **method of cooking** that you are checking for the food.

Remember also that all food composition tables are only approximate, at best. Foods such as meat can vary a lot from sample to sample; even fruit and vegetables that look and taste alike differ enormously in their vitamin C and mineral content, depending on the conditions of growing and storage.

Dairy produce

To use these tables, see page 85

	Kilocalories	Kilojoules	Carbohydrate	Protein	Fat	Fiber	Calcium	Iron	Vitamin A	Vitamin C	Riboflavin	Thiamine	Niacin
Butter, unsalted, 1 oz (30g)	210	880	0		●				●				
salted, regular, 1 oz (30g)	210	880	0		●				●				
whipped, 1 oz (30g)	210	880	0		●				●				
American (processed) cheese, 1 oz (30g)	100	420	1	○	●		●		●		○		○
American cheese food, 1 oz (30g)	90	380	2	○	●		●		●		○		○
Babybel, 1 oz (30g)	90	380	0	○	●		●		○		○		○
Bel Paese, 1 oz (30g)	80	330	0	○	●		●		○		○		○
Brie, 1 oz (30g)	85	360	0	○	●		●		○		○		○
Boursin, garlic and herbs, 1 oz (30g)	110	460	0		●		○		●				
with pepper, 1 oz (30g)	110	460	0		●		○		●				
Cream cheese, 1 oz (30g)	120	500	0		●		○		●				
Cottage cheese, dry curd, 1 oz (30g)	25	100	1	○	○		○				○		○
creamed, 1 oz (30g)	30	120	1	○	○		○				○		○
Camembert, 1 oz (30g)	85	360	0	○	●		●		○		○		○
Cheddar, domestic, 1 oz (30g)	110	460	0	○	●		●		●		○		○
English, 1 oz (30g)	110	460	0	○	●		●		●		○		○
Cheshire, 1 oz (30g)	110	460	0	○	●		●		●		○		○
Caerphilly, 1 oz (30g)	100	420	0	○	●		●		●		○		○
Danbo, 1 oz (30g)	95	400	0	○	●		●		○		○		○
Danish blue, 1 oz (30g)	100	420	0	○	●		●		●		○		○
Double Gloucester, 1 oz (30g)	100	420	0	○	●		●		●		○		○
Edam, 1 oz (30g)	85	360	0	●	●		●		○		○		○
Elbo, 1 oz (30g)	90	380	0	○	●		●		○		○		○
Emmenthal, 1 oz (30g)	110	460	0	●	●		●		●		○		○
Esrom, 1 oz (30g)	90	380	0	○	●		●		○		○		○
Gorgonzola, 1 oz (30g)	100	420	0	○	●		●		●		○		○
Gouda, 1 oz (30g)	85	360	0	●	●		●		○		○		○
Gruyère, 1 oz (30g)	130	540	0	○	●		●		●		○		○
Havarti, 1 oz (30g)	130	540	0	○	●		●		●		○		○
Leicester, 1 oz (30g)	110	460	0	○	●		●		●		○		○
Limburger, 1 oz (30g)	100	420	1	○	●		●		●		○		○
Mozzarella, 1 oz (30g)	95	400	0	○	●		●		○		○		○
Munster, 1 oz (30g)	100	420	1	○	●		●		●		○		○
Parmesan, 1 oz (30g)	120	500	0	●	●		●		○		○		●
Port Salut, 1 oz (30g)	90	380	0	○	●		●		●		○		○
Ricotta, 1 oz (30g)	70	290	0		●		○		○				
Roquefort, 1 oz (30g)	100	420	0	○	●		●		●		○		○
St Paulin, 1 oz (30g)	90	380	0	○	●		●		○		○		○
Sage Derby, 1 oz (30g)	110	460	0	○	●		●		●		○		○
Samsoe, 1 oz (30g)	90	380	0	○	●		●		○		○		○
Stilton, blue, 1 oz (30g)	130	540	0	○	●		●		●		○		○
Swiss, domestic, 1 oz (30g)	110	460	1	○	●		●		●		○		○
Wensleydale, 1 oz (30g)	110	460	0	○	●		●		●		○		○

Dairy produce
continued

	Kilocalories	Kilojoules	Carbohydrate	Protein	Fat	Fiber	Calcium	Iron	Vitamin A	Vitamin C	Riboflavin	Thiamine	Niacin
Cream, heavy, 1 oz (30 g)	130	550	1		●				●				
light, 1 oz (30 g)	55	230	1		●		○		○				
Eggs, large, raw (1)	85	360	0	○	●		○		●		●	○	●
yolk	70	290	0	○	●		○		●		○	○	○
white	15	65	0	○							○		
boiled	85	360	0	○	●		○		●		●	○	●
poached	85	360	0	○	●		○		●		●	○	●
fried	150	630	0	○	●		○		●		●	○	●
scrambled (2)	360	1500	0	○	●		○		●		●	○	●
Eggs, standard, raw (1)	80	330	0	○	●		○		●		●	○	●
yolk	65	270	0	○	●		○		●		○	○	○
white	15	65	0	○							○		○
boiled	80	330	0	○	●		○		●		●	○	●
poached	80	330	0	○	●		○		●		●	○	●
fried	130	540	0	○	●		○		●		●	○	●
scrambled (2)	340	1400	0	○	●		○		●		●	○	●
Eggs, small, raw (1)	75	310	0	○	●		○		●		●	○	●
yolk	65	270	0	○	●		○		●		○	○	○
white	10	40	0	○							○		○
boiled	75	310	0	○	●		○		●		●	○	●
poached	75	310	0	○	●		○		●		●	○	●
fried	130	540	0	○	●		○		●		●	○	●
scrambled (2)	320	1350	0	○	●		○		●		●	○	●
Half-and-half, 1 oz (30 g)	40	170	1		●		○		○				
Margarine, standard, 1 oz (30 g)	210	880	0		●				●				
diet, 1 oz (30 g)	95	400	0		●				●				
soft-spread, 1 oz (30 g)	210	880	0		●				●				
polyunsaturated, 1 oz (30 g)	210	880	0		●				●				
Milk, whole, 1 fl oz (30 ml)	20	85	1		●		○				○		
skim, 1 fl oz (30 ml)	10	40	1				○				○		
low-fat, 1 fl oz (30 ml)	15	65	2	○			○				○		
human, 1 fl oz (30 ml)	20	85	2		●					○			
powdered, whole, 1 oz (30 g)	140	590	11	○	●		●		●	○	●	○	○
nonfat, regular, 1 oz (30 g)	100	420	15	●			●			○	●	○	●
nonfat, instant, 1 oz (30 g)	100	420	15	●			●			○	●	○	●
goat's, 1 fl oz (30 ml)	20	85	1		●		○						
buttermilk, 1 fl oz (30 ml)	10	40	1				○				○		
condensed, sweetened, whole, 1 fl oz (30 ml)	120	500	21	○	○		●		○		○		○
evaporated, unsweetened, 1 fl oz (30 ml)	45	190	3	○	●		●		○		○		○
Yogurt, whole-milk, 1 oz (30 g)	20	85	2	○			○				○		
5 oz (150 g)	90	380	9	○			●				○		
low-fat, 1 oz (30 g)	15	65	2				○				○		
5 oz (140 g)	75	310	9				●				○		

Meat, poultry and game

*All meat off bone unless otherwise specified.
Cooked weights given unless otherwise specified.*

To use these tables, see page 85

	Kilocalories	Kilojoules	Carbohydrate	Protein	Fat	Fiber	Calcium	Iron	Vitamin A	Vitamin C	Riboflavin	Thiamine	Niacin
Bacon, raw, 2 rashers, 3½oz (100g)	670	2800	1	○	●							○	○
broiled or fried, 2oz (60g)	370	1600	2	○	●							○	○
Canadian, raw, 3 rashers, 3oz (90g)	180	750	0	○	●			○			○	○	○
broiled or fried, 2oz (60g)	170	750	0	○	●			○			○	○	○
Beef, steak, raw, 1oz (30g)	55	230	0	○	●			○			○		●
grilled, 8oz (230g) raw	440	1850	0	●	●			●			○		●
fried, 8oz (230g) raw	500	2100	0	●	●			○			○		●
roast, raw, 1oz (30g)	80	330	0	○	●			○					○
roasted, 3oz (90g)	300	1250	0	●	●			○			○		●
boiled, 3oz (90g)	280	1150	0	●	●			○			○		●
corned, 1oz (30g)	60	250	0	○	●			○					●
ground, lean, raw, 1oz (30g)	35	150	0	○	○			○					●
ground, fatty, raw, 1oz (30g)	65	270	0	○	●			○					●
dried, 1oz (30g)	70	290	0	●	●			○					●
pastrami, 1oz (30g)	70	290	0	●	●			○			○		●
dripping, 1oz (30g)	250	1050	0		●								
stock cube (5), 1oz (30g)	60	250	6	●			○	●					
stock cube (1)	10	40	1										
Bologna, 1oz (30g)	85	360	0	○	●			○			○	○	○
Brains, all kinds, raw, 1oz (30g)	30	130	0	○	●			○		●	○		○
boiled, 4oz (110g)	140	590	0	○	●			○		●	○		○
Braunschweiger, 1oz (30g)	90	380	1	●	●		●	●			●	○	○
Capicola, 1oz (30g)	140	590	0	●	●			○			○	○	○
Chicken, raw, 1oz (30g)	35	150	0	○	○								●
roasted, 4oz (110g)	170	710	0	●	○							○	●
grilled, 4oz (110g)	170	710	0	●	○							○	●
fried, 4oz (110g)	190	790	0	●	●							○	●
boiled, 4oz (110g)	210	880	0	●	○			○				○	●
smoked and roast, 4oz (110g)	170	710	0	●	○							○	●
canned in aspic, 4oz (110g)	230	960	0	●	●			○				○	●
stock cube (5), 1oz (30g)	60	250	6	●			○	○					
(1)	10	40	1										
Duck, raw, 1oz (30g)	120	500	0	○	●			○					○
roast, 4oz (110g)	380	1600	0	●	●			○					○
grilled, 4oz (110g)	380	1600	0	●	●			○					○
fried, 4oz (110g)	400	1650	0	●	●			○					○
smoked and roast, 4oz (110g)	380	1600	0	●	●			○					○
Frogs' legs, raw, 1oz (30g)	20	85	0	○									○

	Kilocalories	Kilojoules	Carbohydrate	Protein	Fat	Fiber	Calcium	Iron	Vitamin A	Vitamin C	Riboflavin	Thiamine	Niacin
fried in butter, 1 oz (30g)	85	360	0	○	●								○
Goose, raw, 1 oz (30g)	65	270	0	○	●			○					○
roast, 3 oz (90g)	270	1150	0	●	●			○					○
Guinea-hen, on bone, roast, 1 lb (450g) raw	490	2050	0	●	●			○			○	○	●
grilled, 1 lb (450g) raw	490	2050	0	●	●			○			○	○	●
Ham, boiled, 3 oz (90g)	230	960	0	●	●			○				○	○
smoked or grilled, 3 oz (90g)	190	790	0	●	●			○			●	●	●
roast, boiled, 3 oz (90g)	230	960	0	●	●			○				○	○
baked, 3 oz (90g)	230	960	0	●	●			○				○	○
canned, 1 oz (30g)	35	150	0	○	○			○			○	●	○
prosciutto, 1 oz (30g)	65	270	0	○	●							●	●
Parma ham, 1 oz (30g)	65	270	0	○	●							●	●
Heart, beef, raw, 1 oz (30g)	30	130	0	○	○			○			●		●
braised, 4 oz (110g)	210	880	1	●	○			●			●	○	●
calf, raw, 1 oz (30g)	35	150	1	○	●			○			●		●
braised, 4 oz (110g)	240	1000	2	●	●			●			●	○	●
lamb, raw, 1 oz (30g)	45	190	0	○	●			○			●		●
braised, 4 oz (110g)	290	1200	1	●	●			●			●	○	●
Kidney, all types, raw, 1 oz (30g)	25	100	0	○	○			●	○	○	●	●	●
fried, 4 oz (110g)	180	750	0	●	○			●	○	○	●	●	●
grilled, 4 oz (110g)	150	630	0	●	○			●	○	○	●	●	●
Lamb, roast, raw, 1 oz (30g)	70	290	0	○	●			○			○		
roasted, 3 oz (90g)	230	960	0	●	●			○			○		
boiled (stewed neck, lean only) 3 oz (90g)	210	880	0	●	●			○			○		○
chop, raw, 6 oz (170g) with bone	530	2200	0	●	●			○			○	○	●
grilled, 6 oz (170g)	400	1650	0	●	●			○			○	○	●
fried, 6 oz (170g)	430	1800	0	●	●			○			○	○	●
Lard, 1 oz (30g)	250	1050	0		●								
Liver, all types, raw, 1 oz (30g)	50	210	0	○	●			●	●	○	●	○	●
fried, 4 oz (110g)	260	1100	4	●	●			●	●	●	●	○	●
Liver sausage, 1 oz (30g)	90	380	1	○	●			●	●		●	○	○
Luncheon meat, 3 oz (90g)	270	1150	5	○	●								○
Mortadella, 1 oz (30g)	85	360	0	●	●			○			○		
Oxtail, raw, 1 oz (30g)	50	210	0	●	●			○			○		
Pâté, chicken liver, 1 oz (30g)	95	400	0	○	●			○	●	○	●		○
duck, 1 oz (30g)	95	400	0	○	●			○			○		
game, 1 oz (30g)	95	400	0	○	●						○		○
goose liver, 1 oz (30g)	110	460	0	○	●			○	●	○	●		●
Pheasant, roast, 12 oz (340g) raw	330	1400	0	●	○		○	●			○		●
Pork, roast, raw, 1 oz (30g)	75	310	0	○	●						○	●	●
roasted, 1 oz (30g)	240	1000	0	●	●			○			○	●	●
chop, raw, 6 oz (170g) with bone	470	1950	0	●	●			○			○	●	●
grilled, 6 oz (170g)	330	1400	0	●	●			○			○	●	●

	Kilocalories	Kilojoules	Carbohydrate	Protein	Fat	Fiber	Calcium	Iron	Vitamin A	Vitamin C	Riboflavin	Thiamine	Niacin
Pork chop, fried, 6oz (170g)	350	1450	0	●	●			○			○	●	●
filet, raw, 1oz (30g)	40	170	0	○	●						○	●	●
grilled, 3oz (90g)	160	670	0	●	○			○			○	●	●
fried, 3oz (90g)	180	750	0	●	●			○			○	●	●
smoked, 1oz (30g)	80	330	0	○	●			○			○	●	●
crackling, 1oz (30g)	180	750	0	○	●								○
suckling pig, roast, 3oz (90g)	340	1400	0	○	●							○	○
Quail, grilled (2), 1lb (450g) raw	330	1400	0	●	●			●					●
fried, 1lb (450g) raw	430	1800	0	●	●			●	○				●
roast, 1lb (450g) raw	330	1400	0	●	●			●					●
Rabbit, raw, 1oz (30g)	35	150	0	○	○						○		●
roast, 4oz (110g)	170	710	0	●	●			○			○		●
grilled, 4oz (110g)	170	710	0	●	●			○			○		●
fried, 4oz (110g)	190	790	0	●	●			○			○		●
boiled, 4oz (110g)	200	840	0	●	○			○			○		●
Salami, 1oz (30g)	140	590	1	●							○	○	●
Sausages, beef, raw, 1oz (30g)	85	360	3	○	●								●
fried, 2oz (60g) raw	110	460	6	○	●		○	○			○		
grilled, 2oz (60g) raw	110	460	6	○	●		○	○			○		
baked, 2oz (60g) raw	110	460	6	○	●		○	○			○		
boiled, 2oz (60g) raw	170	710	7	○	●		○	○			○		
pork, raw, 1oz (30g)	100	420	3	○	●			○					○
fried, 2oz (60g) raw	130	540	5	○	●		○	○			○		
grilled, 2oz (60g) raw	130	540	5	○	●		○	○			○		
baked, 2oz (60g) raw	130	540	5	○	●		○	○			○		
boiled, 2oz (60g) raw	210	880	5	○	●		○	○			○		●
bratwurst, raw, 1oz (30g)	80	330	1	○	●			○					○
boiled, 4oz (110g)	310	1300	3	○	●			○					○
cocktail sausages, canned (3), 1oz (30g)	80	330	1	○	●			○					○
knockwurst, 1oz (30g)	80	340	1	○	●			○			○	○	○
liverwurst, 1oz (30g)	85	360	1	○	●			●	●		●	○	○
sausagemeat, pork, raw, 1oz (30g)	100	420	3	○	●			○					○
beef, 1oz (30g)	85	360	3	○	●			○					●
veal-and-pork, 1oz (30g)	95	400	3	○	●			○					○
Squab, raw, 1oz (30g)	80	340	0	○	●			○					●
Suet, 1oz (30g)	250	1050	0		●								
Sweetbreads, beef, raw, 1oz (30g)	60	250	0	○	●						●	○	○
braised, 4oz (110g)	360	1500	0	○	●						●	○	○
calf, raw, 1oz (30g)	25	110	0	○	○						●	○	○
braised, 4oz (110g)	190	780	0	○	○						●	○	○
lamb, raw, 1oz (30g)	35	150	0	○	●			○			●	○	○
braised, 4oz (110g)	260	1100	6	●	●			○			●	○	○
Tongue, beef, raw, 1oz (30g)	60	260	0	○	●				○		○		●

Meat, poultry and game
continued

	Kilocalories	Kilojoules	Carbohydrate	Protein	Fat	Fiber	Calcium	Iron	Vitamin A	Vitamin C	Riboflavin	Thiamine	Niacin
braised, 4oz (110g)	270	1100	0	●	●			○			○		●
lamb, raw, 1oz (30g)	55	230	0	○	●			○	○	○	○		○
boiled, 1oz (30g)	80	330	0	○	●			○	○	○	○		●
Tripe, raw, 1oz (30g)	15	65	0	○	○		○						○
boiled, 4oz (110g)	110	460	0	○	●		○			○			○
Turkey, raw, 1oz (30g)	30	130	0	○									●
roasted, 4oz (110g)	160	670	0	●				○			○		●
grilled, 4oz (110g)	160	670	0	●				○			○		●
fried, 4oz (110g)	180	750	0	●	○			○			○		●
boiled, 4oz (110g)	210	880	0	●				○			○		●
Veal, roast, raw, 1oz (30g)	30	130	0	○	○			○			○		●
roasted, 4oz (110g)	260	1100	0	●	●			○			○		●
chop, raw, 6oz (170g) with bone	150	630	0	●	○			○			○	○	●
grilled, with added fat, 6oz (170g)	240	1000	0	●	●			○			○		●
fried, 6oz (170g)	240	1000	0	●	○			○			○		●
escalope, raw, 4oz (110g)	120	500	0	●	○			○			○		●
fried in breadcrumbs, 5oz (140g) cooked	300	1250	6	●	○			○			○		●
fried, 4oz (110g) raw	190	790	0	●	●			○			○		●
grilled, with added fat, 4oz (110g) raw	190	790	0	●	●			○			○		●
Venison, raw, 1oz (30g)	40	170	0	○	○			●				○	○
roast, 3oz (90g)	170	710	0	●	○			●				○	○
fried, 3oz (90g)	190	790	0	●	○			●				○	○
grilled, 3oz (90g)	170	710	0	●	○			●				○	○

Seafood

*All fish off bone or shelled
unless otherwise specified.
Cooked weights given
unless otherwise specified.*

	Kilocalories	Kilojoules	Carbohydrate	Protein	Fat	Fiber	Calcium	Iron	Vitamin A	Vitamin C	Riboflavin	Thiamine	Niacin
Abalone, raw, 1oz (30g)	30	130	1	○				○			○		
steamed, 1oz (30g)	25	100	1	○				○			○		
canned, 1oz (30g)	25	100	1	○				○			○		
fried, 1oz (30g)	35	150	1	○	○			○			○		
Anchovy, raw, 1oz (30g)	55	230	0	○	●			○			○		●
canned in oil, 1oz (30g)	55	230	0	○	●			○			○		●
canned in brine, 1oz (30g)	55	230	0	○	●			○			○		●
Bass, raw, 1oz (30g)	25	100	0	○	○								●
steamed, 5oz (140g)	190	790	0	●	○								●
fried, no breadcrumbs, 5oz (140g)	240	1000	0	●	●								●
Bluefish, raw, 1oz (30g)	35	150	0	●	○						○		●
baked, 5oz (140g)	220	920	0	●	○						○		●
fried, 5oz (140g)	290	1200	6	●	●						○		●
Carp, raw, 1oz (30g)	25	100	0	○	○								●

	Kilocalories	Kilojoules	Carbohydrate	Protein	Fat	Fiber	Calcium	Iron	Vitamin A	Vitamin C	Riboflavin	Thiamine	Niacin
Carp, steamed, 5oz (140g)	190	790	0	●									●
fried, no breadcrumbs, 5oz (140g)	240	1000	0	●	●								●
Caviar, red, 1oz (30g)	60	250	0	●	●			○		●	●	○	○
black, 1oz (30g)	60	250	0	●	●			○		●	●	○	○
gray, 1oz (30g)	60	250	0	●	●			○		●	●	○	○
Clam, raw, 1oz (30g)	20	85	0	○	○		○	●					○
steamed, 1oz (30g)	30	130	0	○	○		●	●					○
canned, 1oz (30g)	30	130	0	○	○		●	●					○
Cod, raw, 1oz (30g)	20	85	0	●									○
steamed, 5oz (140g)	130	540	0	●									○
fried, no breadcrumbs, 5oz (140g)	180	750	0	●	○								○
deep-fried in batter, 6oz (170g)	340	1400	13	●	●		○						●
dried, salted, 1oz (30g)	35	150	0	●			●						○
Cod's roe, fried, 1oz (30g)	55	230	1	○	●			○	○	●	●	●	○
smoked, 1oz (30g)	30	130	0	○				○	○	●	●	●	○
Crab, cooked, 1oz (30g)	35	150	0	○	○			○					○
canned, 1oz (30g)	25	100	0	○				○					○
Crayfish (3), 6oz (170g) in shells	70	290	0	○			○	○					○
shelled, 2oz (60g)	60	250	0	○			○	○					○
Eel, raw, 1oz (30g)	50	210	0	○	●				●		○	○	○
steamed, 5oz (140g)	280	1150	0	●	●			○	●		○	○	●
fried, 5oz (140g)	340	1400	0	●	●			○	●		○	○	●
deep-fried in batter, 6oz (170g)	350	1450	7	●	●		○	○	●		○	○	●
smoked, 1oz (30g)	55	230	0	○	●				●		○		○
Flounder, baked, 5oz (140g)	280	1200	0	●	●		○						●
Haddock, raw, 1oz (30g)	20	85	0	○									●
steamed, 5oz (140g)	140	590	0	●			○				○		●
fried in breadcrumbs, 6oz (170g)	300	1250	6	●	●		○	○					○
smoked, raw, 1oz (30g)	20	85	0	○									○
steamed, 5oz (140g)	140	590	0	●			○	○				○	●
Hake, raw, 1oz (30g)	20	85	0	○	○								○
poached, 5oz (140g)	150	630	0	●	○								●
Halibut, raw, 1oz (30g)	25	100	0	○	○								●
poached, 5oz (140g)	190	790	0	●	○								●
fried, no breadcrumbs, 5oz (140g)	240	1000	0	●	●								●
Herring filet, raw, 1oz (30g)	65	270	0	○	●							○	●
steamed, 5oz (140g)	280	1150	0	●	●			○				○	●
fried, 5oz (140g)	330	1400	2	●	●		○	○				○	●
salted, 1oz (30g)	80	330	0	○	●							○	●
pickled, 1oz (30g)	80	330	0	○	●							○	●
roe, fried, 1oz (30g)	70	290	1	○	●			○			○	○	○

	Kilocalories	Kilojoules	Carbohydrate	Protein	Fat	Fiber	Calcium	Iron	Vitamin A	Vitamin C	Riboflavin	Thiamine	Niacin
Kipper filet, frozen, 1oz (30g)	80	330	0	○	●						○		●
steamed, 5oz (140g)	290	1200	0	●	●		○	○			○		●
fried, no breadcrumbs, 5oz (140g)	340	1400	0	●	●		○	○			○		●
Lobster, whole, boiled, 1lb (450g)	190	790	0	●	○		●	●			○	●	●
Mackerel, raw, 1oz (30g)	65	270	0	○	●						○		●
steamed, 5oz (140g)	380	1600	0	●	●			○	○		○	○	●
fried, 5oz (140g)	270	1150	0	●	●			○			○		●
smoked, 5oz (140g)	440	1850	0	●	●			○	○		○		●
Mullet, raw, 1oz (30g)	40	170	0	○	●						○		●
steamed, 5oz (140g)	250	1050	0	●	●			○			○	○	●
fried, no breadcrumbs, 5oz (140g)	300	1250	5	●	●		○	○			○		●
Mussel, raw (6), 3oz (90g)	55	230	0	○	○		○	●					○
steamed, 3oz (90g)	55	230	0	○	○		○	●					○
canned, 3oz (90g)	55	230	0	○	○		○	●					○
Octopus, raw, 1oz (30g)	20	85	0										○
steamed, 5oz (140g)	120	500	0	●								○	○
fried, no breadcrumbs, 5oz (140g)	160	670	0	●	○								●
deep-fried in batter, 6oz (170g)	340	1400	13	●	●		○						●
Oyster, raw (6), 3oz (90g)	45	190	0	○			○	●					○
canned, 3oz (90g)	45	190	0	○			○	●					○
smoked, 3oz (90g)	45	190	0	○			○	●					○
Pike, blue, raw, 1oz (30g)	25	100	0	●									●
Pompano, raw, 1oz (30g)	45	190	0	●	●						○	○	○
Red snapper, raw, 1oz (30g)	25	100	0	●							○		●
Salmon, raw, 1oz (30g)	50	210	0	○	●						○		●
steamed, 5oz (140g)	280	1150	0	●	●						○		●
fried, no breadcrumbs, 5oz (140g)	330	1400	0	●	●			○			○		●
smoked, 1oz (30g)	40	170	0	○	○						○		●
canned, 1oz (30g)	45	190	0	○	●		○	○	○		○		●
Salmon trout, raw, 1oz (30g)	50	210	0	○	●							○	●
poached, 5oz (140g)	280	1150	0	●	●							○	●
Sardine, raw, 1oz (30g)	45	190	0	○	●		●	○			○		●
canned in oil, drained, 1oz (30g)	60	250	0	○	●		●	○			○		●
canned in tomato sauce, 1oz (30g)	50	210	0	○	●		●	●			○		●
Scallop, raw (2), 3oz (90g)	90	380	0	●			○	○					○
steamed, 3oz (90g)	90	380	0	●			○	○					○
fried, 3oz (90g)	110	460	0	●	○		○	○					○
Shrimp in shells, 6oz (170g)	65	270	0	○			○	○					○
shelled, 2oz (60g)	60	250	0	○			○	○					○
boiled, 1oz (30g)	30	130	0	○			○	○					○

Seafood
continued

To use these tables,
see page 85

	Kilocalories	Kilojoules	Carbohydrate	Protein	Fat	Fiber	Calcium	Iron	Vitamin A	Vitamin C	Riboflavin	Thiamine	Niacin
Shrimp, deep-fried in breadcrumbs, 1oz (30g)	90	380	8	○	●		○	○					○
deep-fried in batter, 1oz (30g)	55	230	2	○	●		○						○
Skate, raw, 1oz (30g)	20	85	0	○									○
steamed, 5oz (140g)	130	540	0	●									○
Skate, fried, no breadcrumbs, 5oz (140g)	180	750	0	●	○								○
deep-fried in breadcrumbs, 6oz (170g)	300	1250	6	●	●	●	○	○					○
deep-fried in batter, 6oz (170g)	340	1400	13	●	●	●							●
Smelt, raw, 1oz (30g)	25	100	0	○	○								●
fried, 4oz (110g)	500	2100	0	●	●	●	●	●					○
Sole, lemon, raw, 1oz (30g)	25	100	0	○									○
steamed, 5oz (140g)	130	540	0	●								○	●
fried in breadcrumbs, 6oz (170g)	370	1550	16	●	●	●	○	○					○
Squid, raw, 1oz (30g)	20	85	0	●									○
steamed, 5oz (140g)	120	500	0	●								○	○
fried, no breadcrumbs, 5oz (140g)	170	710	0	●	●							○	○
deep-fried in batter, 5oz (140g)	280	1150	11	●	●	●	○						●
Swordfish, raw, 1oz (30g)	35	150	0	○	●			○	●				●
broiled, 5oz (140g)	240	1000	0	○	●			○	●				●
Trout, raw (1), 8oz (230g)	200	840	0	○	●		○	○					○
steamed, 8oz (230g) raw	200	840	0	○	●		○	○					○
fried, 8oz (230g) raw	300	1250	0	●	●		○	○					○
smoked, 8oz (230g)	200	840	0	●	○		○	○					○
Tuna, canned in oil, 1oz (30g)	80	330	0	○	●			○					●
Turbot, raw, 1oz (30g)	20	85	0	○									●
steamed, 5oz (140g)	140	590	0	●			○				○		●
fried in breadcrumbs, 6oz (170g)	300	1250	6	●	●	●	○	○					●
Weakfish, raw, 1oz (30g)	35	150	0	○	●								○
broiled, 5oz (140g)	290	1200	0	●	●								○
Whitefish, raw, 1oz (30g)	45	190	0	●	●					●		○	○
smoked, 1oz (30g)	45	190	0	●	●					●		○	○
Whiting, raw, 1oz (30g)	30	130	0	○	○								○

Vegetables

	Kilocalories	Kilojoules	Carbohydrate	Protein	Fat	Fiber	Calcium	Iron	Vitamin A	Vitamin C	Riboflavin	Thiamine	Niacin
Artichoke, globe, boiled (1), 8oz (230g)	15	65	3							○			
heart, boiled, 4oz (110g)	15	65	3							○			
canned, 4oz (110g)	15	65	3							○			
frozen, 1oz (30g)	7	30	2							○			
Artichoke, Jerusalem, boiled, 4oz (110g)	20	85	4										

Vegetables
continued

	Kilocalories	Kilojoules	Carbohydrate	Protein	Fat	Fiber	Calcium	Iron	Vitamin A	Vitamin C	Riboflavin	Thiamine	Niacin
Asparagus, raw, 1oz (30g)	3	15	0							●			
steamed, 4oz (110g)	10	40	1							○			
canned, 4oz (110g)	10	40	1							○			
frozen, 1oz (30g)	8	35	1							●			
Avocado (½), raw, 4oz (110g)	250	1050	2		●			○		●			○
Bamboo shoots, canned, 1oz (30g)	8	35	1										
Beans, baked, canned (2tbs), 1½oz (45g)	25	100	4			●	○	○					○
broad, raw, 1oz (30g)	15	65	2				○	○		●			○
boiled, 4oz (110g)	55	230	8				○	○		●			○
kidney, dried, 1oz (30g)	95	400	18	○		○	○	●			○	●	○
dried, cooked, 4oz (110g)	130	550	24	○			○	○				○	
canned, 1oz (30g)	25	100	5	○			○	○				○	
lima, raw, 1oz (30g)	35	150	6	○			○	○		●		○	○
cooked, 4oz (110g)	120	500	22	○			○	○		●		○	○
canned, 1oz (30g)	30	130	5	○				○		○			
dried, 1oz (30g)	100	420	18	○			○	●			○	○	○
dried, cooked, 4oz (110g)	150	630	29	○			○	●			○	○	○
frozen, 1oz (30g)	30	130	6	○			○	○		●			○
snap, green, raw, 1oz (30g)	9	40	2				○	○	○	●			
boiled, 4oz (110g)	30	130	6				○	○	○	●			
canned, 1oz (30g)	8	35	2				○	○	○	○			
frozen, 1oz (30g)	8	35	2				○		○	○			
snap, yellow or wax, raw, 1oz (30g)	8	35	2				○	○	○	●			
boiled, 4oz (110g)	25	100	5				○	○	○	○			
canned, 1oz (30g)	8	35	2				○	○	○	○			
frozen, 1oz (30g)	8	35	2				○		○	○			
Beansprouts, raw, 1oz (30g)	3	15	0				○		○				
2oz (60g)	6	25	1				○		○				
boiled, 4oz (110g)	10	40	1				○		○				
Beets, boiled, small, ½oz (15g)	6	25	1				○			○			
medium, 2oz (60g)	25	100	6				○			○			
large, 4oz (110g)	50	210	11				○			○			
pickled, small, ½oz (15g)	6	25	1				○			○			
Broccoli, raw, 1oz (30g)	7	25	1				○	○	○	●	○		
boiled, 4oz (110g)	20	85	2				○	○	●	●	○		
frozen, 1oz (30g)	7	30	1				○	○	○	●	○		
Brussels sprouts, raw, 1oz (30g)	7	30	1				○			●			
boiled, 4oz (110g)	20	85	2	○		●	○	○	○	●	○	○	○
frozen, 1oz (30g)	7	30	1				○			●			
Cabbage, Chinese, raw, 1oz (30g)	4	15	1							●			
boiled, 4oz (110g)	10	40	2							●			
stir-fried, 4oz (110g)	80	330	3		●					●			

	Kilocalories	Kilojoules	Carbohydrate	Protein	Fat	Fiber	Calcium	Iron	Vitamin A	Vitamin C	Riboflavin	Thiamine	Niacin
Cabbage, red, raw, 1 oz (30 g)	6	25	1			○				●			
boiled, 4 oz (110 g)	15	65	3			○				●			
cooked in wine, apples and sugar, 4 oz (110 g)	40	170	9			○				●			
pickled, 1 oz (30 g)	6	25	1			○				●			
Savoy, raw, 1 oz (30 g)	7	30	1			○	○			●			
boiled, 4 oz (110 g)	10	40	1			○	○			●			
white, raw, 1 oz (30 g)	6	25	1			○				●			
boiled, 4 oz (110 g)	15	65	3			○				●			
common, raw, 1 oz (30 g)	6	25	1			○	○			●			
boiled, 4 oz (110 g)	15	65	3			○				●			
Capers, 1 oz (30 g)	0	0	0										
Carrots, raw, 1 oz (30 g)	7	25	2			○			●	○			
boiled, 4 oz (110 g)	20	85	5			○			●	○			
spring, raw, 1 oz (30 g)	7	30	2			○			●	○			
boiled, 4 oz (110 g)	25	100	5			○			●	○			
canned, 1 oz (30 g)	5	20	1			○		○	●				
juice, 1 fl. oz (30 ml)	7	25	2						●	○			
Cauliflower, raw, 1 oz (30 g)	4	15	0							●			
boiled, 4 oz (110 g)	10	40	1							●			
frozen, 1 oz (30 g)	4	15	0							●			
pickled, 1 oz (30 g)	3	10	0							●			
Celeriac, raw, 1 oz (30 g)	7	30	1			○	○			○			
boiled, 4 oz (110 g)	15	65	2			○	○			○			
Celery, raw, 1 oz (30 g)	2	9	0			○				○			
boiled, 4 oz (110 g)	6	25	1			○	○			○			
Chicory, raw, 1 oz (30 g)	3	10	0							○			
boiled, 1 oz (30 g)	2	6	0										
Corn on the cob, raw, 5 in (13 cm), 5 oz (140 g)	180	750	34			○		○	●				○
boiled, 5 oz (140 g)	170	710	32			○		○		○			○
frozen, 1 ear, 5 oz (140 g)	180	760	34			○		○		○			○
Corn oil, 1 fl. oz (30 ml)	250	1050	0		●								
Cucumber, raw, 1 oz (30 g)	3	10	1							○			
pickled, 1 oz (30 g)	3	10	1										
Eggplant, raw, 1 oz (30 g)	4	15	1			○				○			
fried in oil, 4 oz (110 g)	140	590	4		●	○				○			
Endive, raw, 1 oz (30 g)	3	15	0			○		○	●	●			
boiled, 4 oz (110 g)	10	40	1					○	●	●			
Garlic, 1 clove, raw	1	5	0										
Gherkin, pickled, small (1)	1	2	0										
medium (1)	2	8	0									○	
Horseradish, raw, grated, 1 tsp	2	7	0							●			
Horseradish sauce, fresh ½ oz (15 g)	30	130	4		●					●			

	Kilocalories	Kilojoules	Carbohydrate	Protein	Fat	Fiber	Calcium	Iron	Vitamin A	Vitamin C	Riboflavin	Thiamine	Niacin
Kale, raw, 1oz (30g)	15	65	3			○	●	○	●	●	○	○	○
boiled, 4oz (110g)	35	150	6			○	○	○	●	●	○	○	○
frozen, 1oz (30g)	15	65	3			○	○	○	●	●	○	○	○
Kohlrabi, raw, 1oz (30g)	7	30	1				○	○		●			
boiled, 4oz (110g)	10	40	1				○	○		●			
Leeks, raw, 1oz (30g)	9	35	2				○	○	○	●			
boiled, 4oz (110g)	25	100	5				○	○	○	●			
Lentils, dried, 1oz (30g)	85	360	15	○		●		●			○	●	○
boiled, 4oz (110g)	110	460	19	○			○	○				○	○
Lettuce, raw, 1oz (30g)	3	15	0		○	○			○	●			
2oz (60g)	7	30	1		○	○			○	●			
Mushrooms, raw, 1oz (30g)	4	15	0			○					○		○
boiled, 3oz (90g)	7	30	0			○					○		○
fried, 3oz (90g)	180	750	0		●	○		○			○		○
canned, 1oz (30g)	2	9	0										○
Mustard greens, 1oz (30g)	3	10	0			○	○		○	●			
Okra, raw, 1oz (30g)	5	20	1			○	○			●			
boiled, 4oz (110g)	20	85	3			○	○	○		●			
canned, 4oz (110g)	20	85	3			○	○	○		●			
frozen, 1oz (30g)	5	20	1			○	○			●			
Olives, black with pits (10), 1oz (30g)	25	100	0		●	○							
green with pits (10), 1oz (30g)	25	100	0		●	○							
stuffed (10), 1oz (30g)	30	130	0		●	○							○
Olive oil, 1fl.oz (30ml)	250	1050	0		●								
Onions, raw, 1oz (30g)	7	25	1							○			
boiled, 4oz (110g)	15	65	3							○			
baked, 4oz (110g)	25	100	6							○			
fried, 1oz (30g)	100	420	3		●	○	○						
pickled, 1oz (30g)	7	25	1										
Palm heart, canned, 1oz (30g)	30	130	8										
Parsley, raw, 1oz (30g)	6	25	0			●	●	●	●	●	○	○	
Parsnips, raw, 1oz (30g)	15	65	3				○	○		●			
boiled, 4oz (110g)	65	270	15				○			○			
Peas, raw, 1oz (30g)	20	85	3				○	○		●		○	○
boiled, 4oz (110g)	60	250	9				○	○		●		○	○
canned, 1oz (30g)	15	65	2				○	○		●			○
frozen, 1oz (30g)	20	85	3				○	○		●		○	○
Peppers, raw, 1oz (30g)	4	20	1		○					●			
Potatoes, raw, 1oz (30g)	25	100	6							●			
boiled, 4oz (110g)	90	380	22							○			
baked (1), 2½in (6cm) diameter	110	460	26			○				○			○
mashed with milk and butter, 4oz (110g)	130	540	20		○					○			
new, raw, 1oz (30g)	25	100	6							●		○	○

	Kilocalories	Kilojoules	Carbohydrate	Protein	Fat	Fiber	Calcium	Iron	Vitamin A	Vitamin C	Riboflavin	Thiamine	Niacin
Potatoes, boiled, 4 oz (110g)	85	360	21							●		○	○
French fries, thin-cut, 4 oz (110g)	360	1500	42	●				○		○			○
thick-cut, 4 oz (110g)	180	750	31	○						○			○
crinkle-cut, 4 oz (110g)	360	1500	42	●				○		○			○
croquettes (2), 4 oz (110g)	200	840	25	●						○			
sautéed in butter, 4 oz (110g)	200	840	22	●					○	○			
roast with fat, 4 oz (110g)	180	750	31	○						○			○
chips, 1 oz (30g)	150	630	14	●	●			○		●		○	○
packet, 2 oz (60g)	300	1250	28	●	●			○		●		○	○
dried, mixed with water, 4 oz (110g)	80	330	18			○				○			○
mixed with milk, 4 oz (110g)	140	590	22	○	○	○				○	○		○
Pimientos, canned, 1 oz (30g)	8	35	2					○	●	●			
Pumpkin, raw, 1 oz (30g)	4	20	1					○	○				
boiled, 4 oz (110g)	7	30	2			○			●	○			
Radishes, 1 oz (30g)	4	15	1					○		●			
Salsify, raw, 1 oz (30g)	5	20	1			○	○						
boiled, 4 oz (110g)	20	85	3			○	○						
Sauerkraut, canned, 4 oz (110g)	20	85	4			○				●			
Shallots, raw, 1 oz (30g)	7	30	1							○			
Split peas, dried, 1 oz (30g)	90	380	16	○		●		●			○	●	○
boiled, 4 oz (110g)	130	540	25	○		○		○				○	○
Spinach, raw, 1 oz (30g)	10	40	0			●	●	●	●	●			○
boiled, 4 oz (110g)	35	150	2			●	●	●	●	●			○
canned, 1 oz (30g)	8	35	0			○	●	●	●	●			○
frozen, 1 oz (30g)	10	40	0			○	●	●	●	●			○
Squash, summer, raw, 1 oz (30g)	5	20	1						○	●			
boiled, 4 oz (110g)	15	65	3						○	○			
winter, raw, 1 oz (30g)	15	65	4			○			●	○			
boiled, 4 oz (110g)	45	190	10			○			●	○			
Sweetcorn, canned, 1 oz (30g)	20	85	5			○				○			
Sweet potatoes, raw, 1 oz (30g)	25	100	6			○			●	●			
boiled, 4 oz (110g)	95	400	23			○			●	●			
Swiss chard, raw, 1 oz (30g)	7	30	1				○	○	●	●	○		
boiled, 4 oz (110g)	20	85	4				○	○	●	●			
Tomato, raw, 1 oz (30g)	4	15	1						○	●			
medium (1), 1¼in (3cm) diameter, 4 oz (110g)	15	65	3						○	●			
canned, 1 oz (30g)	3	15	1						○	●			
sauce, not bottled, 1 oz (30g)	25	100	2	●					○	○			
ketchup, 1 oz (30g)	30	130	7					○					
purée, 1 oz (30g)	20	85	3					●	●	●		○	○
juice, 1 fl oz (30ml)	5	20	1						○	●			
Turnips, raw, 1 oz (30g)	6	25	1			○	○			●			
boiled, 4 oz (110g)	15	65	3				○			●			

Vegetables
continued

	Kilocalories	Kilojoules	Carbohydrate	Protein	Fat	Fiber	Calcium	Iron	Vitamin A	Vitamin C	Riboflavin	Thiamine	Niacin
Vegetable shortening, 1 oz (30 g)	250	1050	0		●								
Water chestnuts, canned, 1 oz (30 g)	15	65	4							○			
Watercress, raw, 3 oz (90 g)	10	40	1			○	○	○	●	●			
Yeast, fresh, 1 oz (30 g)	15	65	0	○		○		●			●	●	●
dried, 1 oz (30 g)	50	210	1	●		●	○	●			●	●	●
Zucchini, raw, 1 oz (30 g)	3	10	1						○				
boiled, 4 oz (110 g)	5	20	1						●				
fried, 4 oz (110 g)	140	590	2		●				○				
frozen, 1 oz (30 g)	3	15	1						○				

Fruit, nuts and seeds

	Kilocalories	Kilojoules	Carbohydrate	Protein	Fat	Fiber	Calcium	Iron	Vitamin A	Vitamin C	Riboflavin	Thiamine	Niacin
Almonds, shelled, raw, 1 oz (30 g)	160	670	1	○	●	●	●	●			●	○	○
roasted and salted, 1 oz (30 g)	170	710	1	○	●	●	●	●			●	○	○
marzipan, 1 oz (30 g)	65	270	18			○	○						
Angelica, 1 oz (30 g)	80	330	21										
Apple, small, raw, 4 oz (110 g)	40	170	10										
medium, 6 oz (170 g)	50	210	13										
large, 8 oz (230 g)	80	330	21			○				○			
stewed, no sugar, 5 oz (140 g)	45	190	12			○				●			
dried, 1 oz (30 g)	65	270	17			●		○			○		
sauce, unsweetened, 1 oz (30 g)	15	65	3							○			
sweetened, 1 oz (30 g)	20	85	5							○			
juice, natural, 1 fl. oz (30 ml)	10	40	3							○			
½ pint (3 dl)	100	420	27							○			
sweetened, 1 fl. oz (30 ml)	15	65	4							○			
½ pint (3 dl)	160	670	42							○			
Apricot, raw (1)	9	40	2			○			●	○			
stewed, no sugar, 5 oz (140 g)	35	150	8						○	○			
dried (2), 1 oz (30 g)	50	210	12			●	○	●	●		○		○
soaked, stewed, no sugar, 5 oz (140 g)	110	460	28			●		○	○				○
canned in medium syrup (½), 1 oz (30 g)	30	130	8						○				
jam, 1 oz (30 g)	75	310	20						○				
Banana, small, 4½ oz (135 g)	60	250	15			○				○			
medium, 5 oz (140 g)	65	270	16			○				○			
large, 7 oz (200 g)	95	400	23			○				○			
dried, 1 oz (30 g)	65	270	16			●		○	○		○		○
Blackberries, raw, 1 oz (30 g)	8	35	2			●	○			●			
stewed, 5 oz (140 g)	35	150	8			●	○	○		●			
canned in syrup, 1 oz (30 g)	15	65	4			○				●			
jam, 1 oz (30 g)	75	310	20					○		○			

	Kilocalories	Kilojoules	Carbohydrate	Protein	Fat	Fiber	Calcium	Iron	Vitamin A	Vitamin C	Riboflavin	Thiamine	Niacin
Black currants, raw, 1 oz (30g)	8	35	2			●	○	○		●			
canned in medium syrup, 1 oz (30g)	20	85	6			○				●			
jam or jelly, 1 oz (30g)	75	310	20					○		●			
Blueberries, raw, 1 oz (30g)	20	85	4			○		○		○			
frozen, 1 oz (30g)	20	85	4			○		○		○			
Brazil nuts, shelled, 1 oz (30g)	180	750	1	○	●	●	○	○				●	○
Citron, 1 oz (30g)	85	360	22										
Cashew nuts, shelled, 1 oz (30g)	160	670	8	○	●			○			○	○	○
roasted and salted, 1 oz (30g)	150	630	5	○	●			○			○	○	○
packet, 4 oz (110g)	610	2550	18	○	●			○			○	○	○
Cherries, raw, 1 oz (30g)	10	40	3						○				
stewed, no sugar, 5 oz (140g)	55	230	14						○				
candied, 1 oz (30g)	60	250	16					○					
Cherries, canned, 1 oz (30g)	20	85	5										
jam, 1 oz (30g)	75	310	20										
Chestnuts, shelled, raw, 1 oz (30g)	50	210	10			○					○	○	
dried, 1 oz (30g)	95	400	20			●	○	○			○	○	
soaked, boiled, 1 oz (30g)	50	210	10			○					○	○	
roast, with shells, 1 oz (30g)	45	190	9			○					○	○	
Clementine, 2 oz (60g)	20	85	5			○	○			●		○	
Coconut, shelled, raw, 1 oz (30g)	100	420	1		●	●		○					
desiccated, 1 oz (30g)	170	710	2		●	●		○					
milk, 1 fl.oz (30ml)	6	25	1										
cream, 1 oz (30g)	90	380	2		●			○					
Cranberries, raw, 1 oz (30g)	4	20	1			○		○		●			
sauce or jelly, 1 oz (30g)	40	170	10										
Currants, dried, 1 oz (30g)	70	290	18			○	○	○					
Dates, with pits, 1 oz (30g)	60	250	16			●	○	○					○
pitted, 1 oz (30g)	70	290	18			●	○	○					○
Fig, raw (1), 1½ oz (45g)	15	65	4			○		○					
dried (1), ¾ oz (22g)	45	190	11			●	●	○					
soaked, stewed, 5 oz (140g)	170	710	42			●	●	○					
canned in medium syrup, 1 oz (30g)	40	170	10			●	○	○					
Ginger root, raw, 1 oz (30g)	15	65	3										
candied, 1 oz (30g)	100	420	27										
Gooseberries, raw, 1 oz (30g)	5	20	1			○				●			
stewed, no sugar, 5 oz (140g)	20	85	4			○				●			
canned, 1 oz (30g)	40	170	10			○	○	○		●			
Grapefruit, raw (½), 7 oz (200g)	20	85	5							●			
canned, 1 oz (30g)	15	65	4							●			
juice, unsweetened, 1 fl.oz (30ml)	9	35	2							●			
7 fl.oz (200ml)	60	250	16							●			

	Kilocalories	Kilojoules	Carbohydrate	Protein	Fat	Fiber	Calcium	Iron	Vitamin A	Vitamin C	Riboflavin	Thiamine	Niacin
sweetened, 1fl.oz (30ml)	10	40	3							●			
7fl.oz (200ml)	70	310	19							●			
Grapes, black, without stems (6), 1oz (30g)	15	65	4							○			
white, without stems (6), 1oz (30g)	15	65	4							○			
juice, 1fl.oz (30ml)	20	85	5							○			
½ pint (3dl)	180	750	46				○			○			
Greengage, raw, with stones, 1oz (30g)	15	65	3						○				
stewed, no sugar, 5oz (140g)	55	230	14						○	○			
jam, 1oz (30g)	75	310	20										
Hazelnuts, shelled, 1oz (30g)	110	460	2	●	○		○					○	○
Jam, any flavor, 1oz (30g)	75	310	20										
Kumquats, raw (1)	10	40	3			○		○		●			
Lemon, raw, 3oz (90g)	15	65	3			○	○			●			
juice, unsweetened, 1fl.oz (30ml)	2	8	0							●			
Lime, raw (1), 3oz (90g)	20	85	6							●			
juice, unsweetened, 1fl.oz (30ml)	8	35	3							●			
Loganberries, raw, 1oz (30g)	5	20	1			○		○		●			
canned in medium syrup, 1oz (30g)	30	130	7			○		○		●			
Lichees, raw, 1oz (30g)	20	85	5							●			
canned, 1oz (30g)	20	85	5							○			
Macadamia nuts, raw, shelled, 1oz (30g)	200	840	16	○	●	○	○					○	
Mandarin, medium, raw (1), 2½oz (75g)	25	100	6				○	○		●		○	
canned in medium syrup, 1oz (30g)	15	65	4							●			
Mango, raw, 7oz (200g)	120	500	30			○			●	●			
chutney, 1oz (30g)	55	230	14							○			
Melon, cantaloupe, 6oz (170g)	25	100	6					○	●	●			
honeydew, 6oz (170g)	20	85	5							●			
watermelon, 6oz (170g)	20	85	5							○			
yellow, 6oz (170g)	20	85	5						●				
Mulberries, raw, 1oz (30g)	10	40	2					○		○			
canned in medium syrup, 1oz (30g)	25	100	6					○		○			
Mustard, powder, 1oz (30g)	130	540	6	○	●		●	●					
prepared, 1 tsp	10	40	0		●								
Nectarine, with pit, raw, 5oz (140g)	65	270	16			○			○	○			
Nuts and raisins, 4oz (110g)	480	1900	41	○	●	●	○	○				●	●
Orange, medium, raw (1), 3in (7½cm) diameter	60	250	14			○	○			●		○	
juice, 1fl.oz (30ml)	9	40	2							●			

Fruit, nuts and seeds
continued

To use these tables, see page 85

	Kilocalories	Kilojoules	Carbohydrate	Protein	Fat	Fiber	Calcium	Iron	Vitamin A	Vitamin C	Riboflavin	Thiamine	Niacin
Orange juice, ½ pint (3dl)	95	400	24					○		●		○	
sweetened, 1 fl.oz (30ml)	15	65	4							●			
½ pint (3dl)	140	590	36							●	○		
Marmalade, 1oz (30g)	75	310	20							○			
Papaya, raw, 1oz (30g)	10	40	3						●	●			
Passion fruit, raw, 4oz (110g)	15	65	3			○				○			
Peach, medium, raw (1), 2in (5cm) diameter	35	150	9						○	○			
dried, 1oz (30g)	60	250	15			●		●	●		○		○
soaked, stewed, 5oz (140g)	110	460	28			○		○	○				○
canned in medium syrup, 1oz (30g)	50	210	13						○	○			
jam, 1oz (30g)	75	310	20						○				
Peanuts, shelled, 1oz (30g)	160	670	2	○	●	●	○	○				●	●
with shells, 1oz (30g)	110	460	2	○	●	○		○				●	●
shelled and roasted, 1oz (30g)	160	670	2	○	●	●	○	○			○		●
4oz (110g)	650	2700	10	●	●								●
Peanut butter, 1oz (30g)	180	750	4	○	●	●					○		●
Pear, medium (1), 6½oz (195g)	55	230	14			○				○			
canned in medium syrup (½), 2oz (60g)	45	190	11			○							
Pecans, raw, shelled, 1oz (30g)	190	800	4	○	●	●	○	○				●	
Persimmon, raw (1), 1oz (30g)	30	130	8			○		○	●				
Pineapple, raw, 1oz (30g)	15	65	3							●			
canned in medium syrup, 1oz (30g)	20	85	6							●			
candied, 1oz (30g)	85	360	22							●			
juice, unsweetened, 1 fl.oz (30ml)	15	65	4							○			
5 fl.oz (140ml)	75	310	19							○			
jam, 1oz (30g)	75	310	20							○			
Pinenuts (Pignolias), 1oz (30g)	160	670	3	●	●							●	
Pistachio nuts, shelled, raw, 1oz (30g)	170	710	5	○	●			○	●			●	
roasted and salted, 1oz (30g)	170	710	5	○	●			○	●			●	
Plums, large, raw (2), 4oz (110g)	40	170	10							○			
stewed, no sugar, 1oz (30g)	6	25	1			○							
canned in medium syrup, 1oz (30g)	15	65	4							○			
jam, 1oz (30g)	75	310	20										
damsons, 1oz (30g)	10	40	2			○							
stewed, no sugar, 5oz (140g)	45	190	11			○				○			
Pomegranate, raw (1), 7oz (200g)	75	310	20							●			
juice, unsweetened, 1 fl.oz (30ml)	10	40	3							○			
½ pint (3dl)	120	500	33							●			
Prunes, dried, with pits, 1oz (30g)	40	170	9			●			○	○			

Fruit, nuts and seeds
continued

	Kilocalories	Kilojoules	Carbohydrate	Protein	Fat	Fiber	Calcium	Iron	Vitamin A	Vitamin C	Riboflavin	Thiamine	Niacin
soaked, stewed, no sugar, 5oz (140g)	100	420	26			●		○	○				
canned in medium syrup, 1oz (30g)	25	100	7			○		○					
juice, unsweetened, 1fl.oz (30ml)	20	85	5					○					
½ pint (3dl)	220	920	54					○					
Raisins, 1oz (30g)	70	290	18			○	○	○					
Raspberries, raw, 1oz (30g)	7	30	2			●		○		●			
5oz (140g)	35	150	8			●	○	○		●			
canned in medium syrup, 1oz (30g)	25	100	6			○		○		○			
jam, 1oz (30g)	75	310	20					○		○			
Red currants, raw, 1oz (30g)	6	25	1			●		○		●			
stewed, 5oz (140g)	25	100	5			●		○		●			
jelly or jam, 1oz (30g)	75	310	20					○		○			
Rhubarb, raw, 1oz (30g)	2	7	0			○	○			○			
stewed, no sugar, 5oz (140g)	8	35	1			○	○			○			
canned in medium syrup, 1oz (30g)	15	65	3			○	○			○			
Sesame seeds, 1oz (30g)	160	670	6	○	●	○	●	●			○	●	○
oil, 1fl.oz. (30ml)	250	1050	0		●								
Strawberries, raw, 1oz (30g)	10	4	2					○		●			
frozen, sweetened, 1oz (30g)	30	130	8					○		●			
Sunflower oil, 1fl.oz (30ml)	250	1050	0		●								
Tangerine, medium, raw (1), 3oz (90g)	20	85	5				○	○		●	○		
canned in medium syrup, 1oz (30g)	15	65	4							●			
Walnuts, shelled, 1oz (30g)	150	630	1	○	●	○	○	○			○	○	○
pickled, 1oz (30g)	15	65	3										

Grain products

	Kilocalories	Kilojoules	Carbohydrate	Protein	Fat	Fiber	Calcium	Iron	Vitamin A	Vitamin C	Riboflavin	Thiamine	Niacin
Arrowroot, 1oz (30g)	100	420	27			○		○					
Barley, raw, 1oz (30g)	100	420	24			○							○
Bran, 1oz (30g)	60	250	8	○	○	●	○	●			○	●	●
Bread, banana, 1 slice, 1oz (30g)	90	380	16	○			○	○	○				
Boston brown, 1 slice, 1oz (30g)	55	230	12				○	○	○			○	
cornbread, 1 slice, 1oz (30g)	80	330	11		●		○	○				○	○
cracked wheat, 1 slice, 1oz (30g)	75	320	14	○			○	○	○			○	○ ○
date-nut, 1 slice, 1oz (30g)	75	310	12	○			○	○					○
French, 1½in (3·75cm), 1oz (30g)	80	330	16	○			○	○	○				○ ○

	Kilocalories	Kilojoules	Carbohydrate	Protein	Fat	Fiber	Calcium	Iron	Vitamin A	Vitamin C	Riboflavin	Thiamine	Niacin
Bread, high-protein, 1oz (30g)	65	270	12	○		○	○	○			○	○	○
Italian, 1oz (30g)	85	360	17	○		○	○				○	○	○
pita (1), 3oz (90g)	220	920	51				○	○				○	○
pumpernickel, 1 slice, 1oz (30g)	65	270	13	○		○	○	○				○	○
raisin, 1 slice, 1oz (30g)	70	290	13			○	○	○				○	○
rye, dark, 1 slice, 1oz (30g)	65	270	14			○	○	○				○	○
light, 1 slice, 1oz (30g)	65	270	14	○		●	○	○				○	○
soda, 1 slice, 1oz (30g)	75	310	13	○	○	○	○	○				○	○
sourdough, 1 slice, 1oz (30g)	70	290	13	○			○	○				○	○
toast, 1 slice, 1oz (30g)	65	270	14			○	○	○				○	○
whole-grain, 1 slice, 1oz (30g)	60	250	12	○		●		○				○	○
white, crusty, 1 slice, 1½oz (45g)	100	420	21	○		○	○	○				○	○
soft, 1 slice, 1½oz (45g)	100	420	21	○		○	○	○				○	○
Bread products: bagel, (1), 2oz (60g)	170	710	38	○		○	●	●			○	●	●
biscuits, baking powder, 1oz (30g)	140	590	17	○	●	○	○	○				○	○
buttermilk, 1oz (30g)	120	500	19	○	○	○	●	○				○	○
brioche (1), 2½oz (75g)	220	920	25	○	●	○	●	●	●		○	○	●
cinnamon buns, 4oz (110g)	350	1450	70				○	○				○	○
croissant (1), 2½oz (75g)	260	1100	30		●		○	○	○			○	○
Danish pastry, cheese-filled, 4oz (110g)	410	1700	40	○	●		○	○	○		○	○	○
flapjack (1), 2oz (60g)	220	920	30	○	●	○	●	●				○	○
French toast, 1 slice, 5oz (140g)	330	1400	35	○	●		○	○	○		○		○
hot cross bun (1), 4oz (110g)	310	1300	52		○		○	○				○	○
ice cream cone wafer (1)	25	100	5										
matzo (1), 1oz (30g)	110	460	25	○		○		○					○
muffins, blueberry, 4oz (110g)	360	1500	56		○		○	○	○				○
bran, 4oz (110g)	300	1250	47	○	●	○	●	○			●	○	●
corn, 4oz (110g)	250	1050	41	○	○			○				○	○
English (1), 3oz (90g)	180	750	32		○		○	○				○	○
pancakes, sweet, 5oz (140g)	430	1800	36	○	●		○	○				○	○
popovers, 4oz (110g)	240	1000	21	○	●		○	○				○	○
rolls, cloverleaf (1), 2oz (60g)	140	590	23	○	○	○	●	●	○		○	●	●
crusty (1), 2oz (60g)	160	670	32	○		○	●	●				●	●
parkerhouse (1), 2oz (60g)	180	750	18	○	●	○	●	●	●		○	○	●
soft (1), 2oz (60g)	170	710	30	○	○	○	●	○				●	○
whole-grain (1), 2oz (60g)	130	540	18	○	●	○	○	○			●	●	●
waffles, 2oz (60g)	150	630	10	○	●		○	○	●		○	○	
Cornmeal, white, 1oz (30g)	100	420	22	○				○	○		○	○	○

Grain products
continued

	Kilocalories	Kilojoules	Carbohydrate	Protein	Fat	Fiber	Calcium	Iron	Vitamin A	Vitamin C	Riboflavin	Thiamine	Niacin
yellow, 1oz (30g)	100	420	22	○				○			○	○	
Cornstarch, 1oz (30g)	75	320	25										
Flour, all-purpose, 1oz (30g)	100	420	22	○		○		○			○	○	○
buckwheat, 1oz (30g)	100	420	23			○		○					
cake, 1oz (30g)	100	420	22	○		○	○	○			○	○	○
whole-grain, 1oz (30g)	90	380	19	○		●		●				●	●
Oats, raw, 1oz (30g)	110	460	21	○		○	○	●				●	○
Pasta (all types), cooked, 1oz (30g)	35	150	7										
dry, 1oz (30g)	110	460	23	○			○	○					○
Pastry dough, choux, raw, 1oz (30g)	60	250	6		●			○	○				
baked, 1oz (30g)	95	400	9	○	●			○	○	○			○
flaky, raw, 1oz (30g)	120	500	10		●			○	○	○		○	
baked, 1oz (30g)	160	670	13		●			○	○				○
hot-water crust, raw, 1oz (30g)	100	420	12		●			○				○	○
baked, 1oz (30g)	120	500	14		●	○		○				○	○
puff, raw, 1oz (30g)	120	500	9		●			○		●			
baked, 1oz (30g)	150	630	11		●			○		●		○	○
short crust, plain, raw, 1oz (30g)	130	540	14		●			○	○	○		○	○
baked, 1oz (30g)	150	630	16		●	○		○	○	○		○	○
sweet, raw, 1oz (30g)	130	540	14		●			○	○	○		○	○
baked, 1oz (30g)	150	630	16		●	○		○	○	○		○	○
Popcorn, raw, 1oz (30g)	100	420	20	○		○						●	
popped, plain, 1oz (30g)	110	460	22	○		○						●	
popped, oil and salt, 1oz (30g)	130	550	17	○	●	○						○	
popped, caramel-coated, 1oz (30g)	110	460	24									○	
Rice, white, raw, 1oz (30g)	100	420	25			○							○
boiled, 1oz (30g)	35	150	8										
brown, raw, 1oz (30g)	100	420	24			○							○
boiled, 1oz (30g)	35	150	8										
Tapioca, raw, 1oz (30g)	100	420	27			○							
pudding, 4oz (110g)	150	630	23	○			○						
Wheat germ, 1oz (30g)	100	420	13	○	○	●		●			○	●	●

Miscellaneous

	Kilocalories	Kilojoules	Carbohydrate	Protein	Fat	Fiber	Calcium	Iron	Vitamin A	Vitamin C	Riboflavin	Thiamine	Niacin
Chocolate, baking, 1oz (30g)	150	630	9		●			○					
bittersweet, 1oz (30g)	150	630	18		●			○					
milk, 1oz (30g)	150	630	17	○	●		●	○			○		
semi-sweet morsels, 1oz (30g)	150	630	18		●			○					
syrup, 1fl.oz (30ml)	90	380	24					○					
Corn syrup, dark, 1oz (30g)	85	360	21										

	Kilocalories	Kilojoules	Carbohydrate	Protein	Fat	Fiber	Calcium	Iron	Vitamin A	Vitamin C	Riboflavin	Thiamine	Niacin
Corn syrup, light, 1oz (30g)	80	340	21										
Gelatine, unflavored, 1oz (30g)	95	400	0										
Honey, 1oz (30g)	80	330	22										
Marzipan (synthetic), 1oz (30g)	130	540	14	○	●	○	○	○			○		○
Mincemeat, 1oz (30g)	65	270	18			○		○					
Molasses, dark, 1oz (30g)	65	270	17				●	●					
light, 1oz (30g)	70	290	18				○	●					
Pancake syrup, 1oz (30g)	80	340	21										
Sugar, white, granulated, 1oz (30g)	110	420	30										
confectioner's, 1oz (30g)	110	420	30										
brown, 1oz (30g)	110	420	30				○	○					
Vinegar, 1fl.oz (30ml)	1	5	0										

Homemade desserts

	Kilocalories	Kilojoules	Carbohydrate	Protein	Fat	Fiber	Calcium	Iron	Vitamin A	Vitamin C	Riboflavin	Thiamine	Niacin
Ambrosia, 1 portion, 13oz (390g)	300	1250	51		○	●	○	○		●		○	
Angel food cake, 1 portion, 4oz (110g)	270	1150	64								○		○
Apple pie, 1 portion, 8oz (230g)	620	2600	98	○						●			
10oz (300g) with vanilla ice cream	710	2950	112	○						●			
Apple strudel, 1 portion, 4oz (110g)	170	710	29	○	○			○					
Baked Alaska, 1 portion, 10oz (300g)	640	2700	127				○						
Baked custard, 1 portion, 4oz (110g)	140	590	16	○			○				○		
Banana cream pie, 1 portion, 4oz (110g)	300	1250	25		●		○		○				
Banana fritters, 7oz (200g)	400	1650	49	○	●	○	○	○	○	○	○	○	○
Beignets, 4oz (110g)	370	1550	40	○	●		○	○	○		○	○	○
Blueberry pie, 1 portion, 4oz (110g)	270	1150	43	○					○				
Bread-and-butter pudding, 1 portion, 8oz (230g)	460	1900	62	○	○	○	○	○	○		○	○	○
Brown betty, 1 portion, 6oz (170g)	320	1350	79			○	○	○		●			
Charlotte russe, 1 portion, 4oz (110g)	330	1400	22		●		○	○	○		○		
Cheesecake, 1 portion, 4oz (110g)	410	1700	53		●		○	○	○		○		○
Cherries jubilee, 1 portion, 6oz (170g)	230	960	40				○		○				
Cherry pie, 4oz (110g)	300	1250	45	○									
Chocolate brownies, 4oz (110g)	500	2100	54		●			○	○				
Chocolate cream pie, 1 portion, 4oz (110g)	350	1450	36		●		○	○					
Chocolate éclair, 4oz (110g)	370	1550	63	○			○	○					

Homemade desserts
continued

	Kilocalories	Kilojoules	Carbohydrate	Protein	Fat	Fiber	Calcium	Iron	Vitamin A	Vitamin C	Riboflavin	Thiamine	Niacin
Chocolate mousse, 1 portion, 4oz (110g)	320	1350	24		●			○	○		○		
Chocolate soufflé, 1 portion, 8oz (230g)	470	1950	61	○	●			○	○		○		○
Coconut cream pie, 1 portion, 4oz (110g)	310	1300	43		●		○		○				
Coconut layer cake, 1 portion, 4oz (110g)	290	1200	28		●		○						
Cream puffs, 4oz (110g)	360	1500	58	○					○				
Crêpes suzette, 1 portion, 9oz (270g)	710	2950	67		●				○	●			
Deep-dish peach pie, 1 portion, 4oz (110g)	240	1000	29		●		○		○		○		
Devil's food cake with chocolate frosting, 1 portion, 4oz (110g)	210	880	26		●				○	○			
Donuts, plain, 4oz (110g)	370	1550	55	○			○	○			○	○	
jelly, 4oz (110g)	420	1750	55		●		○	○			○	○	
Fruitcake, dark, 1 portion, 4oz (110g)	310	1300	49	○		○	○	○					
light, 1 portion, 4oz (110g)	430	1800	45	○	●	○	○	○	○		○	○	○
Fruit salad, fresh, 1 portion, 9oz (270g)	130	540	34			○			●				
canned, 4oz (110g)	110	460	28					○	○				
Gingerbread, 1 portion, 4oz (110g)	340	1400	52		○		●	○	○			○	○
Indian pudding, 1 portion, 4oz (110g)	120	500	13		●						○		
Jelly-roll cake, 1 portion, 4oz (110g)	330	1400	74				○		○				
Key lime pie, 1 portion, 4oz (110g)	270	1150	29		●				○				
Lemon meringue pie, 4oz (110g)	370	1550	53		●		○	○	○	○			○
Meringue, 1 portion, 2oz (60g)	170	710	23		●				○				
Mince pie (1), 3oz (90g)	280	1150	47	○				○					
Nesselrode pie, 4oz (110g)	280	1150	25		●		○	○					
Peach Melba, 1 portion, 5oz (140g)	200	840	43				○		○				
Pecan pralines, 1 portion, 3oz (90g)	390	1650	53		●		○						
Pineapple upside-down cake, 1 portion, 4oz (110g)	310	1300	45		●			○					
Pumpkin pie, 1 portion, 4oz (110g)	230	960	25		●		○		○				
Rhubarb pie, 1 portion, 8oz (230g)	560	2350	83		●		○		○				
Rice pudding, 1 portion, 7oz (200g)	260	1100	40	○			●		○		○		○
Rum baba (2 small), 1 portion, 7oz (200g)	500	2100	70	○									
Sacher torte, 1 portion, 4oz (110g)	410	1790	43	○	●		○	○	○		○		○
Sauces, all per oz (30g): butterscotch	140	590	17		●				●				

Homemade desserts
continued

To use these tables, see page 85

	Kilocalories	Kilojoules	Carbohydrate	Protein	Fat	Fiber	Calcium	Iron	Vitamin A	Vitamin C	Riboflavin	Thiamine	Niacin
Sauces, English custard (thin)	35	150	3	●			●		○		●		
fudge	150	630	19	●				○	○		○		
hard (rum or brandy butter)	140	590	12	●					●				
lemon	50	210	9	○									
strawberry	30	130	8							●			
Southern pecan pie, 1 portion, 4oz (110g)	450	1900	47		●			○	○				○
Spice cake, 1 portion, 4oz (110g)	340	1400	58	○				○	○	○			○
Sponge cake, 1 portion, 4oz (110g)	330	1400	65	○				○			○	○	○
Strawberry bavarian cream, 1 portion, 4oz (110g)	220	920	22		●				○	●			
Strawberries with cream and sugar, 5oz (140g)	150	630	23	○						●			
Tapioca pudding, 1 portion, 7oz (200g)	230	960	37	○			●				○		
Trifle, with custard sauce, 6oz (170g)	250	1050	37	○			○	○		○	○		
with cream, 5oz (140g)	240	1000	28		●		○	○		○	○		
Yellow cake with chocolate frosting, 4oz (110g)	420	1750	66	○			○	○	○				

Homemade main dishes, side dishes and accompaniments

	Kilocalories	Kilojoules	Carbohydrate	Protein	Fat	Fiber	Calcium	Iron	Vitamin A	Vitamin C	Riboflavin	Thiamine	Niacin
Artichoke (globe), with butter, 4oz (110g)	50	210	1		●				○				
with vinaigrette, 4oz (110g)	45	190	1		●				○				
Asparagus, with hollandaise, 5oz (140g)	190	790	1		●			○	○	○			
Avocado guacamole, 5oz (140g)	260	1100	3		●			○		●			○
with shrimp and mayonnaise, 4oz (110g)	270	1150	2	○	●			○		●			○
with vinaigrette, 4oz (110g)	350	1450	2		●			○		●			○
Baked beans, 4oz (110g)	70	290	12			●	○	○					
Baked stuffed pork chops, 1 portion, 10oz (300g)	750	3150	30	●	●			○				●	●
Baked Virginia ham, 4oz (110g)	300	1250	0	●	●			○				○	●
Barbecued spare ribs, 1 portion, 14oz (420g)	230	960	36		○		○	○	○	●		○	○
Beef Burgundy, 1 portion, 24oz (700g)	680	2850	12	●	●			●		○	○	○	●
Beef and vegetable stew, 1 portion, 22oz (660g)	770	3200	46	●	●	○	●	●	●	○			●
Beef curry, 1 portion, 14oz (420g)	580	2450	7	○	●			●		●	○		●
with rice, 4oz (110g)	780	3250	57	●	●			●		●	○		●

Homemade main dishes, side dishes and accompaniments
continued

	Kilocalories	Kilojoules	Carbohydrate	Protein	Fat	Fiber	Calcium	Iron	Vitamin A	Vitamin C	Riboflavin	Thiamine	Niacin
Beef stroganoff, 1 portion, 14 oz (420 g)	570	2400	4	○	●			○	○		○		●
Beef wellington, 1 portion, 14 oz (420 g)	1050	4400	57	●	●			○	●		○	○	●
Bouillabaisse, 1 portion, 7 oz (200 g)	260	1100	6	○	●			○		○		○	○
Brunswick stew, 1 portion, 1 lb (450 g)	400	1650	30	●	○	●	○	○	○	○	○	○	●
Calf's liver, sautéed with onions, 1 portion, 1 lb (450 g)	600	2500	27	○	●			●	●	●	●	○	●
Cannelloni, 1 portion, 10 oz (300 g)	760	3200	58	○	●		●	○	○		○		●
Cauliflower, in cheese sauce, 1 portion, 9 oz (270 g)	350	1450	16	○	●	○	●	○	○	○	○		○
Cheese blintzes, 11 oz (330 g)	650	2700	44	●	●		○		○				○
Cheese fondue, 1 portion, 10 oz (300 g)	850	3550	68	●	●		●	○	○		○		●
Cheese soufflé, 1 portion, 4 oz (110 g)	280	1150	8	●	●		●	○	○		○		
Cheese straws, 1 portion (3), 1 oz (30 g)	160	670	9	○	●		●	○	●		○	○	○
Chicken à la King, 1 portion, 14 oz (420 g)	640	2700	10	●	●			○	○	○	●		●
Chicken and dumplings, 1 portion, 12 oz (340 g)	500	2100	27	○	●								●
Chicken cacciatore, 1 portion, 12 oz (340 g)	330	1400	10	●	●			○	○	○	●	○	●
Chicken chasseur, 1 portion, 15 oz (440 g)	360	1500	1	●	●			○	○	○	○	○	●
Chicken curry, 1 portion, 12 oz (340 g)	490	2050	7	●	●		○	●	○		○	○	●
with rice, 4 oz (110 g)	700	2950	57	●	○			●	●		●		●
Chicken fricassée, 1 portion, 20 oz (600 g)	570	2400	10	●	●						○	○	●
Chicken Kiev, 1 portion, 10 oz (300 g)	780	3250	44	○	●				○				●
Chicken livers, sautéed with onions, 1 portion, 8 oz (230 g)	330	1400	13	●	●			●	●	●	●	●	●
Chicken tetrazzini, 1 portion, 22 oz (660 g)	1250	5250	87	●	●		●	○	●		○	○	●
Chili con carne, 1 portion, 11 oz (330 g)	400	1650	19	●	●	○	○	●	○	●	○	○	●
Chop suey, 1 portion, 10 oz (300 g)	270	1150	5	●	●	○	○	○		●	●	●	
Chopped liver, 1 portion, 2½ oz (75 g)	130	540	1	○	●			●	●	○	●	○	○
Chow mein, 1 portion, 13 oz (390 g)	660	2750	99	○									○
Coq au vin, 1 portion, 26 oz (780 g)	810	3400	7	●	●			○	○	●	○	○	●
Coquilles St Jacques, 1 portion, 6 oz (170 g)	240	1000	17	○	●		○	○	○	○	○	○	○
Corn and ham fritters, 9 oz (270 g)	530	2200	65	○	○		○				○	○	
Corned beef hash, 7 oz (200 g)	300	1250	12	●	●			○		●	○		●

109

	Kilocalories	Kilojoules	Carbohydrate	Protein	Fat	Fiber	Calcium	Iron	Vitamin A	Vitamin C	Riboflavin	Thiamine	Niacin
Corn on the cob, with butter, 5oz (140g)	280	1150	32	●	○			○	○	○		○	○
Crab cocktail, 1 portion, 6oz (170g)	450	1990	1	○	●		○	○	○				○
Creamed spinach, 1 portion, 10oz (300g)	270	1150	11	○	●	●	●	●	●	●	○	○	○
Devilled eggs, 5oz (140g)	370	1550	0	●	●		○		○		○		○
Devilled Maryland crab, 1 portion, 12oz (340g)	460	1900	19	●	●		●	○	○	●	○		●
Duck, roast with orange sauce, 1 portion, 18oz (540g)	810	3400	27	○	●		○		●				○
Egg foo yung, 1 portion, 8oz (230g)	320	1350	0	●	●		○	○	○		○	○	○
Eggs à la Russe, 8oz (230g)	740	3100	8	○	●						○		
Eggs Benedict, 10oz (300g)	740	3100	30	○	●		○		●		○	○	○
Garlic bread, 3in (7½cm), 2½oz (75g)	270	1150	32	●	●	○	●	●	●			●	●
Gefilte fish, boiled, 1 portion, 7oz (200g)	180	750	12	●			○	○	●	○	○	○	○
Goulash, 1 portion, 19oz (570g)	750	3150	32	○	●			●	●	○			●
Hamburger, plain, 8oz (230g) raw, 6oz (170g) cooked	450	1900	12	●	●		○	●			○		●
in roll, 2oz (60g)	620	2600	42	○	●			○					●
with French fries, 3oz (90g), pickles, ½oz (15g)	890	3700	72	○	●			●					●
Harvard beets, 5oz (140g)	160	670	31	○						○			
Hot dog in roll, with mustard and relish, 4oz (110g)	350	1450	36	○	●		○	○				○	○
Irish stew, 1 portion, 20oz (600g)	690	2900	51	○	●				●				●
Lamb curry, 1 portion, 14oz (420g)	720	3000	7	○	●			●	●	○			●
with rice, 4oz (110g)	930	3900	57	○	●			●	●	○	○	○	●
Lamb kebabs, 1 portion, 7oz (200g) cooked	660	2750	4	●	●								○
with pita, 3oz (90g)	880	3700	54	○	●			○					●
Lasagne, 1 portion, 1lb (450g)	1200	5000	68	●	●		●	●	●	●	○	○	●
Lobster thermidor, 1 portion, 12oz (340g)	570	2400	6	●	●		●	●	○				●
Macaroni cheese, 1 portion, 14oz (420g)	570	2400	62	●	●		●	●	○				●
Meat loaf, 1 portion, 10oz (300g)	610	2550	25	○	●			●			○	○	●
Moules marinières, 1 portion, 10oz (300g)	310	1300	1	●	●		●	●	○	○			○
Moussaka, 1 portion, 14oz (420g)	730	3050	24	○	●		○	○	○	○	●		●
New England boiled dinner, 1 portion, 15oz (440g)	870	3650	17	●	●			●	○	○	○		●
Noodles Alfredo, 1 portion, 9oz (270g)	870	3650	69	●	●		●	○	●	○			○
Omelet, plain, 1 portion, 5oz (140g)	270	1150	0	○	●		○		○		○		○
cheese, 1 portion, 6oz (170g)	340	1400	0	●	●		●		●		○		○

	Kilocalories	Kilojoules	Carbohydrate	Protein	Fat	Fiber	Calcium	Iron	Vitamin A	Vitamin C	Riboflavin	Thiamine	Niacin
fines herbes, 1 portion, 5oz (140g)	270	1150	0	○	●		○		●	○	○		○
ham, 1 portion, 5oz (140g)	270	1150	0	●	●		○	○	○		○	○	○
mushroom, 1 portion, 5oz (140g)	270	1150	0	○	●		○		○		○		○
Spanish, 1 portion, 8oz (230g)	290	1200	6	○	●		○		○	●	○	○	○
Ossobuco, 10oz (300g)	390	1650	16	●	●		○	○	○	●	○		●
Oysters Rockefeller (6), brown bread, 1oz (30g), butter, lemon	150	630	13	○	○		○	●	○		○		○
Oysters, scalloped, no shells, 5oz (140g)	440	1850	33	○	●		○	●	●	○		○	○
Paella, 1 portion, 20oz (600g)	630	2650	67	●	○			○	●	●			●
Pâté, chicken liver, 2oz (60g), toast, 2oz (60g), butter, ½oz (15g)	470	1950	31	○	●		○	●	●	●	●	○	○
duck, as above	410	1700	31	○	●		○	○		○	○	○	○
goose liver, as above	470	1950	31	○	●		○	○		○	○	○	○
Pizza, 10oz (300g)	660	2750	70	○	●		●	○			○		
Potatoes au gratin, 1 portion, 6oz (170g)	260	1100	22	○	●		○		○	●	○	○	○
Potato pancakes, 6oz (170g)	230	960	27	●	●			○		○	○	○	○
Pot roast with vegetables, 1 portion, 15oz (440g)	550	2300	23	○	●			○	○	●	○		●
Quiche lorraine, 1 portion, 5oz (140g)	490	2050	23	○	●		●	○	○		○	○	○
spinach, 1 portion, 10oz (300g)	760	3200	27	●	●		●	●	●		●		
Ratatouille, 1 portion, 12oz (340g)	200	840	11	○	●	○	○	○	○	●	○		○
Ravioli in tomato sauce, with cheese, 1 portion, 11oz (330g)	540	2250	65	○	○		○	○	○	○		○	●
Red cabbage with apples, 1 portion, 4oz (110g)	85	360	13		○	○				●			
Salad, Caesar, 1 portion, 4oz (110g)	130	540	9	○	●		○	○	○	○	○		
chef's, 1 portion, 11oz (330g)	750	3150	2	○	●		●	○	○	○	○		●
chicken, 1 portion, 7oz (200g)	330	1400	1	●	●			○	○	○	○		●
coleslaw, 1 portion, 4oz (110g)	70	290	6		●	○	○			●			
crab, 1 portion, 6oz (170g)	190	790	1	○	●		○	○	○	○	○	○	○
cranberry mold, 1 portion, 5oz (140g)	190	790	32			○	○		○		○		
ham, 3oz (90g) ham, total 8oz (230g)	160	670	4	●	○	○		○	●	●	○	●	●
lobster, 1 portion, 7oz (200g)	270	1150	1	●	●		○	○	○	○		○	○
macaroni with tuna, 1 portion, 13oz (390g)	1150	4800	46	○	●					●			●
niçoise, 1 portion, 14oz (420g)	340	1400	43		●	○	○	○	○	●		○	○

	Kilocalories	Kilojoules	Carbohydrate	Protein	Fat	Fiber	Calcium	Iron	Vitamin A	Vitamin C	Riboflavin	Thiamine	Niacin
Salad, potato, 1 portion, 9oz (270g)	280	1150	40	●	○			○		●		○	○
spinach and bacon, 1 portion, 9oz (270g)	630	2650	3	●	●		●	○	●	●			○
tomato, 1 portion, 3oz (90g)	75	310	2	●				○	●				
tomato aspic, 1 portion, 6oz (170g)	25	100	6	●				○	●				
tuna, 1 portion, 8oz (230g)	640	2700	1	○	●					○			●
Waldorf, 1 portion, 4oz (110g)	130	540	9	●	●					○			
Salmon croquettes, 8oz (230g)	300	1250	15	●	●		○	○	○	○	○	○	○
Sandwiches with white bread, 3oz (90g), butter, ½oz (15g), cheese, 2oz (60g)	530	2200	42	●	●		●	○					○
club, 10oz (300g)	670	2800	44	○	●		○		○		○	○	●
egg salad, 7oz (200g)	470	1950	29	○	●		○	○	○	○	○	○	○
ham, 1½oz (45g)	350	1450	42	○	●		○	○				○	○
(roast) beef, 1½oz (45g)	390	1650	42	○	●		○	○				○	○
tomato, 3oz (90g)	310	1300	45	○	○	○	○	○	●			○	○
turkey, 8oz (230g)	600	2500	28	○	●								●
Sauces, all per oz (30g): barbecue	20	85	4					○	○	●		○	○
béarnaise	120	500	0	●			○		●				
béchamel	40	170	3	●			○	○					
bordelaise	35	150	2	●									
brown	15	65	1	●									
cheese	55	230	3	●	●		●		○		○		
cranberry	40	170	10										
French dressing	220	920	0		●								
hollandaise	140	590	0	●	●			○	●				
horseradish	65	270	8	●	○	○	○	○	○	●			
mayonnaise	230	960	0		●								
remoulade	180	750	0		●						○		
tartare	140	590	0		●								
tomato	25	100	2					○	○				
tomato ketchup	30	130	7					○					
thousand island dressing	140	590	1		●						○		
vinaigrette	220	920	0		●								
white	45	190	3	●			○	○					
Sauerbraten, 1 portion, 10oz (300g)	620	2600	11	○	●			○				○	●
Sauerkraut, 1 portion, 4oz (110g)	100	420	12	●	○					●			
Scalloped potatoes, 1 portion, 6oz (170g)	140	590	24	○			○			○			
Scampi provençale with rice, 1 portion, 13oz (390g)	580	2450	52	○	●		○			○			○
Shrimp cocktail, 1 portion, 2oz (60g)	140	590	1	●			○			○			

Homemade main dishes, side dishes and accompaniments *continued*

	Kilocalories	Kilojoules	Carbohydrate	Protein	Fat	Fiber	Calcium	Iron	Vitamin A	Vitamin C	Riboflavin	Thiamine	Niacin
Shrimp creole, 20oz (600g)	360	1500	17	●	●	○	●	●	●	●	○	○	●
Shrimp curry, 1 portion, 10oz (300g)	300	1250	7	●	●		●	●	○	●			○
Short ribs of beef, braised, on bone, 1 portion, 1lb (450g)	1100	4600	7	●	●			○					●
Soft-shell crabs, sautéed (1), 3oz (90g)	210	880	11	●	●			○					
Sole, bonne femme, 1 portion, 8oz (230g)	180	750	5	●	○		○	○				○	●
mornay, 1 portion, 12oz (340g)	400	1650	10	●	●		●	○	○	○	○	○	●
florentine, 1 portion, 18oz (540g)	730	3050	19	●	●	○	●	●	●	●	○	○	●
meunière, 1 portion, 5oz (140g)	270	1150	8	●	●			○	○			○	○
Soups: borsch, 1 portion, 12oz (340g)	110	460	4	●	●			○	●				
chicken noodle, 10oz (300g)	55	230	10										
consommé, 10oz (300g)	70	290	1	●									
corn chowder, 1 portion, 10oz (300g)	410	1700	34	○	●	○	○	○	○	○	○	○	○
French onion, 1 portion, 14oz (420g)	370	1550	27	○	●	●	●	○		●	○	○	○
gazpacho, 1 portion, 13oz (390g)	280	1150	18	●	●	○	○	○	○	●		○	○
lentil with ham, 1 portion, 11oz (330g)	360	1500	35	○	●	●	○	●			○	○	○
lobster bisque, 1 portion, 14oz (420g)	480	2000	16	○	●		○	○	●			○	○
New England clam chowder, 1 portion, 13oz (390g)	580	2450	14	○	●		●	●	○				○
minestrone, 1 portion, 1lb (450g)	330	1400	36	○	●	●	○	●	●	●	●	○	○
Manhattan clam chowder, 1 portion, 12oz (340g)	190	790	10	●	●	○	○	●	●	●		○	○
mushroom, 1 portion, 10oz (300g)	210	880	8		●	○	○	○	○	○	○	○	○
oxtail, 10oz (300g)	120	500	14		○		○	○					○
pea (thick), 10oz (300g)	280	1150	34	○	○	○	○	○	○			○	○
tomato, 10oz (300g)	160	670	17		●			○	○				
vichyssoise, 1 portion, 1lb (450g)	450	1900	23		●	○	○	○	●	●		○	○
Southern fried chicken, 1 portion, 10oz (300g)	530	2200	24	○	●								●
Spaghetti, with tomato sauce, 1 portion, 14oz (420g)	510	2150	77		○				○	●			
bolognese, 1 portion, 15oz (440g)	550	2300	77		○				○	●			○
Steak, 8oz (230g) raw, 6oz (170g) cooked, French fries, 5oz (140g)	780	3250	41	●	●			●				○	●
Steak-and-kidney pie, 1 portion, 10oz (300g)	990	4150	32	○	●			○	○				●

Homemade main dishes, side dishes and accompaniments *continued*

To use these tables, see page 85

	Kilocalories	Kilojoules	Carbohydrate	Protein	Fat	Fiber	Calcium	Iron	Vitamin A	Vitamin C	Riboflavin	Thiamine	Niacin
Steak au poivre with cream sauce, 1 portion, 6 oz (170 g) raw, 7 oz (200 g) cooked	740	3100	6	○	●			○	○				●
Steak diane, 1 portion, 8 oz (230 g)	750	3150	0	○	●			○	○		○		●
Steak tartare, 1 portion, 10 oz (300 g)	490	2050	1	●	●	○		●	○	○	○	○	●
Stuffed breast of veal, 1 portion, 10 oz (300 g)	570	2400	36	●	○			○			○		●
Stuffed cabbage rolls, 1 portion, 8 oz (230 g)	150	630	17	○	○	○	○	○	○	●	○	○	○
Stuffing: chestnut, 1 oz (30 g)	40	170	6		○	○							
sage and onion, 1 oz (30 g)	60	250	6		●		○	○	○				
sausage and apple, 4 oz (110 g)	190	790	27		●		○	○					○
Succotash, 1 portion, 4 oz (110 g)	200	840	19		●	○		○	○	○		○	○
Sukiyaki, beef, 1 portion, 1 lb (450 g)	710	2950	33	○	●			○	○	●			●
Swedish meatballs, 10 oz (300 g)	430	1800	15	●	●			○	○		○	○	●
Sweet-and-sour pork, 1 portion, 8 oz (230 g), with rice, 4 oz (110 g)	930	3900	86		●							○	○
Swiss steak, 1 portion, 13 oz (390 g)	570	2400	13	○	●			○		○	○		●
Sweet potato soufflé, 1 portion, 4 oz (110 g)	160	670	24		○				●	○	○		
Teriyaki, beef, 1 portion, 10 oz (300 g)	680	2850	9	○	●			○					●
Trout almandine, 1 portion, 10 oz (300 g)	500	2100	8	○	●								○
Turkey, roast, with bread stuffing and giblet gravy, 1 portion, 10 oz (300 g)	430	1800	36	●			○	○			○	○	●
Tuna-fish casserole, 1 portion, 12 oz (340 g)	730	3050	85	○	○								●
Veal birds, 1 portion, 14 oz (420 g)	700	2950	74	○	○		○	○					●
Veal parmigiana, 1 portion, 14 oz (420 g)	820	3450	29	○	●		●	○	○	○	○		●
Vol-au-vent, chicken-and-mushroom, 1 portion, 10 oz (300 g)	570	2400	30	○	●				○	○			●
Welsh rarebit, 1 portion, 4 oz (110 g)	370	1550	25	○	●		●		○		○		○
Wiener schnitzel, 1 portion, 8 oz (230 g)	490	2050	10	●	●			○			○	○	●
Yorkshire pudding, 4 oz (110 g)	240	1000	29	○	●		○	○			○	○	

Nonalcoholic beverages

	Kilocalories	Kilojoules	Carbohydrate	Protein	Fat	Fiber	Calcium	Iron	Vitamin A	Vitamin C	Riboflavin	Thiamine	Niacin
Apple juice, natural, 1 fl. oz (30 ml)	9	40	2							●			
½ pint (3 dl)	90	380	23							●			
sweetened, 1 fl. oz (30 ml)	20	85	5							○			

	Kilocalories	Kilojoules	Carbohydrate	Protein	Fat	Fiber	Calcium	Iron	Vitamin A	Vitamin C	Riboflavin	Thiamine	Niacin
½ pint (3dl)	190	790	49							●			
Apricot juice, natural, 1 fl.oz (30ml)	7	25	2						○	○			
½ pint (3dl)	35	150	8						○	○			
sweetened, 1 fl.oz (30ml)	15	65	4						○	○			
½ pint (3dl)	85	360	22						○	○			
Carrot juice, natural, 1 fl.oz (30ml)	7	25	2						●	○			
½ pint (3dl)	65	270	15				○	○	●	●		○	○
Chocolate, drinking, powder, 1 oz (30g)	100	420	22					○					○
mixed with milk, ½ pint (3dl)	230	960	22	○	●		●		○	○			○
Cocoa powder, 1 oz (30g)	90	380	3	○	●		○	●			○		●
mixed with milk, ½ pint (3dl)	220	920	15	○	●		●	○	○	○	○	○	○
mixed with milk and sugar, ½ pint (3dl)	250	1050	22	○	●		●	○	○	○	○	○	○
Coffee, instant, powder, 1 oz (30g)	30	130	3	○			○	●					●
black, 1 cup, 7 fl.oz (200ml)	4	15	1									
made with milk, 1 cup, 7 fl.oz (200ml)	130	540	9	●			●		○		○		○
made with milk and sugar, 1 cup, 7 fl.oz (200ml)	160	670	17	●			●		○		○		○
ground beans, black, 1 cup, 7 fl.oz (200ml)	4	15	1									
with milk, 7 fl.oz (200ml)	20	85	2	●								
with milk and sugar, 7 fl.oz (200ml)	50	210	9									
with cream, 7 fl.oz (200ml)	35	150	1	●								
with cream and sugar, 7 fl.oz (200ml)	60	250	8	●								
Cream soda, 1 fl.oz (30ml)	7	25	2									
Ginger ale, 1 fl.oz (30ml)	7	30	2									
Grape juice, natural, 1 fl.oz (30ml)	20	85	5							○		
½ pint (3dl)	180	750	46					○		○		
Grapefruit juice, natural, 1 fl.oz (30ml)	9	35	2							●		
½ pint (3dl)	90	380	22							●		
sweetened, 1 fl.oz (30ml)	10	40	3							●		
½ pint (3dl)	110	460	27							●		
Lemon juice, 1 fl.oz (30ml)	2	8	0							●		
Milk, ½ pint (3dl)	180	750	13	○	●		●		○	○	○		○
Milk shake, chocolate, ½ pint (3dl)	220	920	22	○	●		●		○	○	○		○
strawberry, ½ pint (3dl)	200	840	21	○	●		●		○	○	○		○
coffee, ½ pint (3dl)	200	840	21	○	●		●		○	○	○		○
vanilla, ½ pint (3dl)	200	840	21	○	●		●		○	○	○		○
banana, ½ pint (3dl)	200	840	21	○	●		●		○	○	○		○
made with milk, ice cream, chocolate, ½ pint (3dl)	270	1150	33	○	●		●		○		○		○

To use these tables,
see page 85

	Kilocalories	Kilojoules	Carbohydrate	Protein	Fat	Fiber	Calcium	Iron	Vitamin A	Vitamin C	Riboflavin	Thiamine	Niacin
Milk shake, made with milk, ice cream, banana, ⅓ pint (3dl)	260	1100	32	○	○		●		○		○		○
vanilla, ⅓ pint (3dl)	260	1100	32	○	○		●		○		○		○
coffee, ⅓ pint (3dl)	260	1100	32	○	○		●		○		○		○
strawberry, ⅓ pint (3dl)	260	1100	32	○	○		●		○		○		○
Orange juice, natural, 1 fl. oz (30ml)	9	40	2							●			
½ pint (3dl)	95	400	24					○		●		○	
sweetened, 1 fl. oz (30ml)	15	65	4							●			
½ pint (3dl)	140	590	36							●		○	
Orange drink, concentrated 1 fl. oz (30ml)	30	130	8										
Pear juice, ⅓ pint (3dl)	85	360	22								○		
Pineapple juice, 1 fl. oz (30ml)	15	65	4								○		
Prune juice, 1 fl. oz (30ml)	20	85	5					○					
Soda water, 1 fl. oz (30ml)	0	0	0										
Tomato juice, 1 fl. oz (30ml)	5	20	1							○	●		
5 fl. oz (140ml)	25	100	5							○	●		
Tonic water, 1 fl. oz (30ml)	6	25	2										
Tea, black, 1 cup, 7 fl. oz (200ml)	2	8	0										
Tea, with milk, 7 fl. oz (200ml)	20	85	1		●								
with milk, sugar, 7 fl. oz (200ml)	50	210	9	○									

Alcoholic beverages

	Kilocalories	Kilojoules	Carbohydrate	Protein	Fat	Fiber	Calcium	Iron	Vitamin A	Vitamin C	Riboflavin	Thiamine	Niacin
Absinthe, 1 fl. oz (30ml)	65	270	0										
Advocaat, 1 fl. oz (30ml)	75	310	8	○									
Ale, brown, 1 fl. oz (30ml)	8	35	1										
½ pint (3dl)	80	330	8										
pale, 1 fl. oz (30ml)	9	40	1										
½ pint (3dl)	90	380	6										
Anisette, 1 fl. oz (30ml)	65	270	0										
Apricot brandy, 1 fl. oz (30ml)	70	290	9										
Aquavit, 1 fl. oz (30ml)	65	270	0										
Armagnac, 1 fl. oz (30ml)	65	270	0										
Beer, 1 fl. oz (30ml)	15	65	1										
10 fl. oz (300ml)	130	550	11										○
Benedictine, 1 fl. oz (30ml)	110	460	14										
Bitters, 1 dash	0	0	0										
Black-currant liqueur, 1 fl. oz (30ml)	70	290	9										
Black Velvet, ½ pint (3dl)	140	590	9										
Bloody Mary, 7 fl. oz (200ml)	210	880	4							○	●		
Bourbon, 1 fl. oz (30ml)	65	270	0										
Brandy, 1 fl. oz (30ml)	65	270	0										

Alcoholic beverages
continued

	Kilocalories	Kilojoules	Carbohydrate	Protein	Fat	Fiber	Calcium	Iron	Vitamin A	Vitamin C	Riboflavin	Thiamine	Niacin
Bronx cocktail, 3 fl. oz (90ml)	160	670	3										
Calvados, 1 fl. oz (30ml)	70	290	9										
Campari, 1 fl. oz (30ml)	70	290	4										
Cassis, 1 fl. oz (30ml)	70	290	9										
Champagne, 1 fl. oz (30ml)	20	85	0										
Champagne cocktail, 4 fl. oz (110ml)	100	420	6										
Chartreuse, 1 fl. oz (30ml)	120	500	17										
Cherry brandy, 1 fl. oz (30ml)	70	290	9										
Cider, dry, 1 fl. oz (30ml)	10	40	1										
1 pint (6 dl)	200	840	15					○					
sweet, 1 fl. oz (30ml)	10	40	1										
1 pint (6 dl)	240	1000	24					○					
Cognac, 1 fl. oz (30ml)	65	270	0										
Cointreau, 1 fl. oz (30ml)	95	400	9										
Crème de cacao, 1 fl. oz (30ml)	90	380	8										
Crème de menthe, 1 fl. oz (30ml)	90	380	8										
Daiquiri cocktail, 4 fl. oz (110ml)	220	920	8							○			
Dry Martini cocktail, 2½ fl. oz (75ml)	140	590	1										
Dubonnet, 1 fl. oz (30ml)	45	190	4										
Gin, 1 fl. oz (30ml)	65	270	0										
Grand Marnier, 1 fl. oz (30ml)	90	380	8										
Highball cocktail, 8 fl. oz (230ml)	130	540	0										
Horse's neck cocktail, ½ pint (3 dl)	170	710	13										
Hot toddy, 4 fl. oz (110ml)	130	540	15										
Irish coffee, 4 fl. oz (110ml)	160	670	8	○									
Kirsch, 1 fl. oz (30ml)	65	270	0										
Madeira, 1 fl. oz (30ml)	35	150	1										
Manhattan cocktail, sweet, 3 fl. oz (90ml)	160	670	7										
Maraschino, 1 fl. oz (30ml)	70	290	9										
Marsala, 1 fl. oz (30ml)	40	170	2										
Martini, dry, 2½ fl. oz (75ml)	140	590	1										
sweet, 2½ fl. oz (75ml)	150	630	2										
Martini cocktail, 3 fl. oz (90ml)	200	840	0										
Negroni cocktail, 5½ fl. oz (165ml)	200	840	12										
Old-fashioned cocktail, 2 fl. oz (60ml)	110	460	5										
Ouzo, 1 fl. oz (30ml)	65	270	0										
Pernod, 1 fl. oz (30ml)	70	290	0										
Pink lady cocktail, 5½ fl. oz (165ml)	210	880	0							●			
Pink gin cocktail, 5 fl. oz (140ml)	85	360	6										
Port, 1 fl. oz (30ml)	45	190	3										
Retsina, 1 fl. oz (30ml)	20	85	0										
Rum, white, 1 fl. oz (30ml)	65	270	0										
dark, 1 fl. oz (30ml)	65	270	0										

Alcoholic beverages
continued

To use these tables,
see page 85

	Kilocalories	Kilojoules	Carbohydrate	Protein	Fat	Fiber	Calcium	Iron	Vitamin A	Vitamin C	Riboflavin	Thiamine	Niacin
Rusty nail cocktail, 3 fl.oz (90ml)	210	880	8										
Sangria, 11 fl.oz (330ml)	210	880	14					○		○			
Schnapps, 1 fl.oz (30ml)	65	270	0										
Screwdriver cocktail, 5 fl.oz (140ml)	220	920	8							●			
Sherry, dry, 1 fl.oz (30ml)	35	140	0										
medium, 1 fl.oz (30ml)	35	140	1										
sweet, 1 fl.oz (30ml)	40	170	2										
Sidecar cocktail, 3 fl.oz (90ml)	160	670	6							○			
Singapore sling, 6½ fl.oz (195ml)	270	1140	19							○			
Sloe gin, 1 fl.oz (30ml)	45	190	6										
Snowball cocktail, ½ pint (3dl)	200	840	29										
Stout, 1 fl.oz (30ml)	10	40	1										
½ pint (3dl)	100	420	12										
Strega, 1 fl.oz (30ml)	65	270	0										
Tia Maria, 1 fl.oz (30ml)	90	380	8										
Tom Collins, ½ pint (3dl)	250	1050	15							○			
Vermouth, dry, 1 fl.oz (30ml)	35	140	2										
sweet, 1 fl.oz (30ml)	45	190	4										
Vodka, Martini cocktail, 3 fl.oz (90ml)	160	670	3										
Whiskey sour cocktail, 4½ fl.oz (135ml)	230	1000	15							●			
White lady cocktail, 4 fl.oz (110ml)	220	920	8							●			
Wine, red, dry, 1 fl.oz (30ml)	20	85	0					○					
sweet, 1 fl.oz (30ml)	25	100	1					○					
white, dry, 1 fl.oz (30ml)	20	85	0					○					
medium, 1 fl.oz (30ml)	20	85	1					○					
sweet, 1 fl.oz (30ml)	25	100	2					○					
sparkling, dry, 1 fl.oz (30ml)	20	85	0					○					
medium, 1 fl.oz (30ml)	20	85	1					○					
sweet, 1 fl.oz (30ml)	25	100	2					○					

Brand names

BREAKFAST CEREALS (dry)													
All-Bran (Kellogg), 1 fl.oz (30ml)	70	290	22	○		●		●	●	●	●	●	●
Cheerios (General Mills), 1 oz (30g)	110	460	20	○		●	○	●	●	●	●	●	●
Corn Flakes (Kellogg), 1 oz (30g)	110	460	25	○		●		●	●	●	●	●	●
Corn Pops (Kellogg), 1 oz (30g)	110	460	26			●		●	●	●	●	●	●
Froot Loops (Kellogg), 1 oz (30g)	110	460	25			●		●	●	●	●	●	●
Frosted Flakes (Kellogg), 1 oz (30g)	110	460	26			●		●	●	●	●	●	●
Frosted Mini-Wheats (Kellogg), 1 oz (30g)	110	460	24	○		●		●	●	●	●	●	●
Grape-Nuts Flakes (Post), 1 oz (30g)	100	420	23	○		○		●	●		●	●	●

	Kilocalories	Kilojoules	Carbohydrate	Protein	Fat	Fiber	Calcium	Iron	Vitamin A	Vitamin C	Riboflavin	Thiamine	Niacin
Honey Smacks (Kellogg), 1 oz (30 g)	110	460	25	○		●		●	●	●	●	●	●
Oat Cracklin' Bran (Kellogg), 1 oz (30 g)	110	460	19	○	○	●		●	●	●	●	●	●
Product 19 (Kellogg), 1 oz (30 g)	110	460	24	○		●		●	●	●	●	●	●
Puffed Rice (Quaker), ½ oz (15 g)	60	250	13			●							
Raisin Bran (Kellogg), 1⅓ oz (40 g)	120	500	29	○		●		●	●		●	●	●
Rice Krispies (Kellogg), 1 oz (30 g)	110	460	25				○	●	●	●	●	●	●
Shredded Wheat (Nabisco) (1)	90	380	19	○		●		○					○
Special K (Kellogg), 1 oz (30 g)	110	460	21				○	●	●	●	●	●	●
Total (General Mills), 1 oz (30 g)	110	460	23	○		●	○	●	●	●	●	●	●
Wheaties (General Mills), 1 oz (30 g)	110	460	23	○		●		●	●	●	●	●	●
BREAKFAST CEREALS (cooked)													
Cream of Wheat (Nabisco), 1 oz (30 g) dry	100	420	22	○				●			○	●	○
Farina (Pillsbury) ⅔ cup with water	80	340	17									○	
Grits, quick (Quaker), ¾ oz (22 g) dry	80	340	18					○			○	○	○
Quick Oats (Quaker), 1 oz (30 g) dry	110	460	18	○				○				●	
Wheatena (Standard Milling), 1 oz (30 g) dry	110	460	21	○				○					○
SOUPS (Canned)													
Black bean (Campbell's), 10 oz (300 g)	130	550	22										
Chicken broth (Campbell's), 10 oz (300 g)	50	210	3	●									
Chicken gumbo (Campbell's), 10 oz (300 g)	70	290	10	○									
Chicken noodle (Campbell's), 10 oz (300 g)	90	380	11	○									
Chicken with rice (Campbell's), 10 oz (300 g)	80	340	9	○									
Chunky minestrone (Campbell's), 9½ oz (285 g)	160	670	25	○					●				
Chunky sirloin burger (Campbell's), 9½ oz (285 g)	210	880	21	○	○				○				○
Consommé, beef (Campbell's), 10 oz (300 g)	45	190	4	○									
Cream of mushroom (Campbell's), 10 oz (300 g)	140	630	11	●									
Cream of potato (Campbell's), 10 oz (300 g)	90	380	14	○									
Split pea with ham, bacon (Campbell's), 10 oz (300 g)	210	880	30	○	○								
Vegetable beef (Campbell's), 10 oz (300 g)	90	380	10						○				
SOUPS (dry)													
Chicken noodle (Lipton), 8 oz (230 g)	70	290	9		○								
Chicken rice (Lipton), 8 oz (230 g)	60	250	8		○								

	Kilocalories	Kilojoules	Carbohydrate	Protein	Fat	Fiber	Calcium	Iron	Vitamin A	Vitamin C	Riboflavin	Thiamine	Niacin
Onion mushroom (Lipton), 8oz (230g)	35	140	5	○									
SOUPS (instant)													
Cup-A-Soup, chicken noodle (Lipton), 6oz (170g)	45	190	6	○									
Cup-A-Soup, green pea (Lipton), 6oz (170g)	120	500	20										
Cup-A-Soup, tomato (Lipton), 6oz (170g)	70	290	13										
BEVERAGES (soft drinks)													
Bitter lemon (Schweppes), 10fl.oz (300ml)	140	590	34										
Cherry drink (Hi-C), 6fl.oz (170ml)	95	400	23							●			
Club Soda (Canada Dry), 6fl.oz (170ml)	0	0	0										
Coca-Cola (Coca-Cola), 8fl.oz (230ml)	95	400	24										
Dr Pepper (Dr Pepper), 8fl.oz (230ml)	95	400	24										
Fresca (Coca-Cola), 8fl.oz (230ml)	2	8	0										
Fruit punch (Hawaiian Punch), 6fl.oz (170ml)	90	380	22							●			
Ginger ale (Canada Dry), 6fl.oz (170ml)	65	270	16										
Grape soda (Welch's), 6fl.oz (170ml)	90	380	23										
Pepsi-Cola (Pepsi-Cola), 8fl.oz (230ml)	100	420	26										
Seven-Up (Seven-Up), 8fl.oz (230ml)	95	400	24										
Sprite (Coca-Cola), 8fl.oz (230ml)	95	400	24										
Tab (Coca-Cola), 8fl.oz (230ml)	1	4	0										
Tonic water (Schweppes), 10fl.oz (300ml)	110	460	28										
BEVERAGES (instant)													
Hot cocoa mix (Swiss Miss), 6fl.oz (170ml)	110	460	21										
Iced tea with lemon, sugar (Lipton), 8fl.oz (230ml)	60	250	16										
Lemonade mix (Country Time), 8fl.oz (230ml)	90	380	22							○			
Quik, chocolate (Nestlé), ⅓oz (22g)	70	290	19										
Quik, strawberry (Nestlé), ⅓oz (22g)	80	340	21										
Tang (General Foods), 4fl.oz (110ml)	60	250	14						○	●			
SAUCES													
Brown gravy mix (French's), 2oz (60g)	20	85	3		○								
Chicken gravy (Franco-American), 2oz (60g)	50	210	3		●								

	Kilocalories	Kilojoules	Carbohydrate	Protein	Fat	Fiber	Calcium	Iron	Vitamin A	Vitamin C	Riboflavin	Thiamine	Niacin
Maggi (Nestlé), 1 cube	6	25	0	○									
Tabasco (McIlhenny), ¼tsp	0	0	0	○									
Worcestershire sauce (French's), ½oz (15g)	10	40	2										
SALAD DRESSINGS													
Blue cheese (Wishbone), ½oz (15g)	80	340	1		●								
Deluxe French (Wishbone), ½oz (15g)	50	210	2		●								
Italian (Wishbone), ½oz (15g)	80	340	1		●								
SPREADS													
Apple butter (Smucker's), ½oz (15g)	25	100	6										
Mayonnaise (Hellman's), ½oz (15g)	100	420	0		●								
Mustard (French's), ½oz (15g)	10	40	1		○								
Peanut butter (Skippy), 1oz (30g)	170	710	4	●	●			○					●
Sandwich spread (Hellman's), ½oz (15g)	60	250	2		●								
Tomato ketchup (Heinz), 1oz (30g)	30	8	130					○					
CONVENIENCE FOODS (main dishes)													
Beef dinner (Banquet), 11oz (330g)	310	1300	21	●	○			●		○			○
Beef enchiladas (Swanson), 15oz (440g)	570	2300	72		○				○				
Beef pepper oriental (La Choy), 8oz (230g)	90	380	10										
Beef pie (Banquet), 8oz (230g)	410	1700	41	○	●			●	○				
Beef stew (Stouffer's), 10oz (300g)	310	1300	16	○	●			○	○		○		○
Chicken à la King, with rice (Stouffer's), 9¼oz (285g)	330	1400	38	○	○								○
Chicken divan (Stouffer's), 8½oz (255g)	340	1450	14	○	●		○		○	○	○		○
Chicken pie (Banquet), 8oz (230g)	430	1700	39	○	●			○					○
Corned-beef hash (Libby's), 8oz (230g)	160	670	8	○	●								
Deviled crabs (Mrs Paul's), 3oz (90g)	160	670	18		○	○							
Fish 'n' chips entrée (Swanson), 5oz (140g)	290	1200	25	○	●								
Fish Parmesan (Mrs Paul's), 5oz (140g)	220	920	20	○	●								
Fish sticks (Mrs Paul's) (4), 3oz (90g)	140	630	16	○	○								
French bread pizza (Stouffer's), 5oz (140g)	330	1400	43	○	○		○	○				○	○
Fried clams (Howard Johnson), 3½oz (100g)	280	1200	32	○	○								
Hungry-Man fried-chicken dinner (Swanson), 10¾oz (322g)	650	2750	51	○	●								○
Hungry-Man Salisbury steak dinner (Swanson), 17oz (510g)	870	3650	65	○	●								○
Hungry-Man veal parmigiana (Swanson), 20½oz (615g)	910	3800	70	○	●								

To use these tables, see page 85

	Kilocalories	Kilojoules	Carbohydrate	Protein	Fat	Fiber	Calcium	Iron	Vitamin A	Vitamin C	Riboflavin	Thiamine	Niacin
Meatballs entrée (Swanson), 9¾oz (277g)	330	1400	26	○	●			○					○
Meat-loaf dinner (Banquet), 11oz (330g)	410	1700	29	○	●			○	○	○			○
Shrimp chow mein (La Choy), 8oz (230g)	75	320	11										
Shrimp croquettes (Howard Johnson), 3½oz (100g)	230	970	20	○	●								
Stuffed peppers (Stouffer's), 7¾oz (232g)	230	970	18	○	●								○
Tuna noodle casserole (Stouffer's), 5¾oz (172g)	200	840	18	○	●								○
CONVENIENCE FOODS (starchy)													
Beef flavor (Rice-a-Roni), 1⅓oz (40g) dry	130	550	27									○	
Beef noodle (Hamburger Helper), ⅕pkg	320	1350	26	○	●			○			○	○	○
Beef ravioli (Franco-American), 7½oz (225g)	220	920	36	○	○				○				○
Chicken-flavor stuffing mix (Stove Top), ½cup	170	710	21	○	●		○	○	○		○	●	○
Herb-seasoned stuffing (Pepperidge Farm), 1oz (30g)	110	460	23	○				○			○	○	○
Idaho mashed potatoes, instant (French's), ½cup	120	500	16		●								
Lasagne with meat sauce (Stouffer's), 10½oz (315g)	390	1650	36	○	○		○	○	○		○	○	○
Macaroni-and-cheese entrée (Banquet), 8oz (230g)	280	1200	36	○	○		○		○				
Spaghetti and meatballs with sauce (Franco-American), 7¼oz (217g)	210	880	23	○	○								
"Spaghetti Os" (Franco-American), 7⅞oz (222g)	160	670	31									○	
Spanish rice mix (rice-a-Roni), 1¼oz (37g) dry	120	500	26									○	
White-and-wild-rice mix (Green Giant), 3½oz (100g)	90	380	19					○					
CONVENIENCE FOODS (vegetables)													
Beans with tomato sauce (Campbell's), 8oz (230g)	260	1100	44	○				○					
Broccoli au gratin (Stouffer's), 5oz (140g)	170	710	9				○		●	○			
Candied yams (sweet potatoes) (Mrs Paul's), 4oz (110g)	170	760	44										○
Cauliflower in cheese sauce (Green Giant), 3½oz (100g)	85	360	6		●					●			
Chop suey vegetables (La Choy), 5oz (140g)	55	230	10										
Corn fritters (Mrs Paul's), 4oz (110g)	260	1100	31		●								○
Corn soufflé (Stouffer's), 4oz (110g)	160	670	19		●				○				
Creamed spinach (Birds Eye), 3oz (90g)	60	250	6						●				

	Kilocalories	Kilojoules	Carbohydrate	Protein	Fat	Fiber	Calcium	Iron	Vitamin A	Vitamin C	Riboflavin	Thiamine	Niacin
Fancy mixed Chinese vegetables (La Choy), 5oz (140g)	65	270	2										
Fried eggplant sticks (Mrs Paul's), 3½oz (100g)	260	1100	27		●								
Fried onion rings (Mrs Paul's), 2½oz (75g)	140	630	21		●								
Italian-style vegetables (Birds Eye), 3⅓oz (40g)	45	190	8		○				○	○			
Japanese-style vegetables (Birds Eye), 3⅓oz (40g)	35	140	7						○	○			
New England-style vegetables (Birds Eye), 3⅓oz (40g)	60	250	11						○	○			
Small onions with cream sauce (Birds Eye), 3oz (90g)	100	420	11		●								
Spinach soufflé (Stouffer's) 4oz (110g)	140	590	12		●				○				
DESSERTS (ready-made)													
Apple pie (Sara Lee), 3½oz (100g)	280	1200	34		●					○			
Apple strudel (Pepperidge Farm), 3oz (90g)	250	1050	31		●								
Apple walnut cake (Pepperidge Farm), 1⅓oz (40g)	130	550	20		○								
Banana cake (Sara Lee), 3½oz (100g)	360	1400	55		○								
Blueberry turnovers (Pepperidge Farm) (1)	320	1350	32		●								
Boston cream pie (Mrs Smith's), ⅙ pie	330	1400	52		○								
Chocolate-filled cupcakes (Hostess), 1¾oz (52g)	160	670	30		○								
Chocolate-frosted donuts (Hostess) (1)	130	550	14		●								
Chocolate Mousse Bavarian (Sara Lee), 3½oz (100g)	360	1400	28		●								
Coconut custard pie (Mrs Smith's), ⅙ pie	260	1100	32		●								
Coconut layer cake (Pepperidge Farm), 1⅔oz (50g)	170	760	26		●								
Cool Whip (Birds Eye), 1 tbs	15	65	1		●								
Cream-cheese cake (Sara Lee), 3½oz (100g)	300	1250	30	○	●								
Crumb cake (Hostess) (1)	130	550	22		○								
German chocolate layer cake (Pepperidge Farm), 1⅓oz (40g)	160	670	24		○								
Jelly donuts (Morton's) (1)	170	760	23		●								
Pecan coffee cake (Sara Lee), 3½oz (100g)	410	1700	45		●			○			○		
Pound cake (Sara Lee), 3½oz (100g)	410	1700	48		●			○			○		
Powdered sugar donuts (Hostess) (1)	110	460	15		●								
Pumpkin pie (Banquet), ⅙ pie	210	880	32		○				○				
Reddi Whip, 4tbs	40	170	2		●							●	

	Kilocalories	Kilojoules	Carbohydrate	Protein	Fat	Fiber	Calcium	Iron	Vitamin A	Vitamin C	Riboflavin	Thiamine	Niacin
Strawberry rhubarb pie (Mrs Smith's), ⅙ pie	320	1350	47		●								
Twinkies (Hostess) (1)	140	590	26		○								
DESSERT MIXES													
Angel-food cake (Duncan Hines) (1)	140	590	30										
Brownie (Duncan Hines) (1)	140	590	21		○								
Chocolate pudding (Royal), 5oz (140g)	170	760	33		○		○				○		
Creamy deluxe frosting, vanilla (Betty Crocker), ⅟₁₂ tub	170	710	28		○								
Dream Whip (General Foods), 1 tbs	8	35	1		●								
Easy-mix coffee cake (Aunt Jemima), ⅛ cake	170	710	29		○								
Gingerbread (Dromedary) 2 in (5cm) square	100	420	19										
Golden egg-custard (Jell-O), ½ cup	170	710	24	○	○		○				○		
Pound cake (Dromedary), 1" (2.5cm) slice	320	1350	46		○								
Raspberry gelatin (Jell-O), ½ cup	80	340	19										
Rice pudding (Jell-O), ½ cup	170	760	30		○		○						
Tapioca (Jell-O), ½ cup	170	710	28		○		○						
Vanilla pudding, instant (Jell-O), ½ cup	170	760	30		○		○						
Wild-blueberry muffins (Duncan Hines) (1)	110	460	17		○								
COOKIES													
Brownie chocolate nut (Pepperidge Farm) (3)	170	710	19	○	●								
Butter-flavored (Nabisco) (6)	140	590	20		○			○			○	○	○
Chocolate chip (Pepperidge Farm) (3)	130	550	17		●								
Fig newton (Nabisco) (2)	110	460	23					○			○		
Ginger snap (Sunshine) (5)	120	500	22		○			○					
Irish oatmeal (Pepperidge Farm) (3)	140	630	21	○	●								
Lorna Doone shortbread (Nabisco) (1)	160	670	19		●			○			○	○	
Mallomar (Nabisco) (2)	110	460	18		○								
Marshmallow sandwich (Nabisco) (4)	130	550	24		○						○		
Oreo chocolate sandwich (Nabisco) (3)	140	630	22		○			○					
Peanut-butter wafer (Sunshine) (4)	130	550	16	○	○			○					
Sugar wafers (Sunshine) (3)	130	550	20		○			○					
Vanilla wafers (Sunshine) (9)	140	590	20	○	○			○					
CRACKERS													
Cheez-its (Sunshine), 1oz (30g) (26)	160	670	16	○	●		○	○					

	Kilocalories	Kilojoules	Carbohydrate	Protein	Fat	Fiber	Calcium	Iron	Vitamin A	Vitamin C	Riboflavin	Thiamine	Niacin
Honey grahams (Sunshine) (1)	60	250	0										
Melba toast, plain (Devonshear), 1oz (30g) (6)	100	420	20	○									
Ritz (Nabisco), 1oz (30g) (9)	140	630	18		○			○			○	○	○
Triscuit (Nabisco), 1oz (30g) (7)	140	590	21	○	○			○					○
Waverly crackers (Nabisco), 1oz (30g) (8)	140	590	21		○		○	○			○	○	○
Wheat thins (Nabisco), 1oz (30g) (16)	140	590	19		○			○			○	○	○
Zwieback toast (Nabisco), 1oz (30g) (4)	120	500	21	○	○			○			○	○	○
DRY SNACKS													
Cocktail peanuts (Planter's), 1oz (30g)	170	710	5	●	●								●
Corn chips (Fritos), 1oz (30g)	160	670	16	○	●								
Dry-roasted cashews (Planter's) 1oz (30g)	160	670	9	○	●			●			○		
Dry-roasted sunflower nuts (Planter's), 1oz (30g)	160	670	5	●	●			○			○		●
Mixed nuts (Planter's), 1oz (30g)	160	670	7	○	●			○			○		○
Sesame nut mix (Planter's), 1oz (30g)	160	670	8	○	●			○					●
Tortilla chips (Doritos), 1oz (30g)	140	590	19		○		○		○				
YOGURT													
Blueberry (Dannon), 8oz (230g)	260	1100	49	○			○				○		
Boysenberry (Dannon), 8oz (230g)	260	1100	49	○			○				○		
Cherry (Dannon), 8oz (230g)	260	1100	49	○			○				○		
Coffee (Dannon), 8oz (230g)	200	840	32	○			○				○		
Dutch apple (Dannon), 8oz (230g)	260	1100	49	○			○				○		
Honey-pear (Dannon), 8oz (230g)	260	1100	49	○			○				○		
Lemon (Dannon), 8oz (230g)	200	840	32	○			○				○		
Peach (Dannon), 8oz (230g)	260	1100	49	○			○				○		
Pina Collada (Dannon), 8oz (230g)	260	1100	49	○			○				○		
Plain (Dannon), 8oz (230g)	140	630	17	○			○				○		
Red raspberry (Dannon) 8oz (230g)	260	1100	49	○			○				○		
YOGURT (Frozen)													
Danny-in-a-cup (Dannon), 8fl.oz (230ml)	210	880	42				○				○		
Danny yogurt on-a-stick, strawberry, choc-coated (Dannon), 2½fl.oz (75ml)	130	550	15		●								
ICE CREAM													
Butter pecan (Howard Johnson), 2oz (60g)	160	670	13	○	●								
Cherry vanilla (Howard Johnson), 2oz (60g)	140	590	11	○	●								
Chip crunch (Good Humor), 1⅜oz (50g)	110	460	10		●								
Chocolate (Howard Johnson), 2oz (60g)	140	630	15	○	●								

	Kilocalories	Kilojoules	Carbohydrate	Protein	Fat	Fiber	Calcium	Iron	Vitamin A	Vitamin C	Riboflavin	Thiamine	Niacin
Chocolate chip (Howard Johnson), 4fl.oz (110ml)	160	670	15	○	●								
Chocolate-coated vanilla (Good Humor), 3oz (90g)	170	710	12	○	●		○				○		
Coffee (Howard Johnson), 2oz (60g)	140	590	11	○	●								
Mint chip (Howard Johnson), 4fl.oz (110 ml)	160	670	15	○	●								
Orange sherbet (Howard Johnson), 2oz (60g)	75	310	17										
Raspberry sherbet (Howard Johnson), 2oz (60g)	70	290	14										
Strawberry (Howard Johnson), 2oz (60g)	130	550	13	○	●								
Vanilla (Howard Johnson), 2oz (60g)	140	590	12	○	●								
Whammy, assorted flavors (Good Humor), 1¼oz (45g)	50	210	13										
CANDY AND GUM													
Baby Ruth (Curtiss), 1¾oz (52g)	260	1100	31	○	●						○		○
Bubble Yum (Life Savers Inc), 1 piece	25	100	7										
Butterfinger (Curtiss), 1⅝oz (50g)	220	920	28	○	●			○			○		○
Butterscotch discs (Brach's), 1oz (30g)	110	460	27										
Chocolate-covered peanuts (Goober's), 1oz (30g)	140	630	16										
Chunky (Ward Johnson Inc), 1oz (30g)	140	630	17										
Crunch bar (Nestlé), 1oz (30g)	140	630	18	○	●		○				○		
$100,000 bar (Nestlé), 1oz (30g)	140	590	19	○							○		
Life Savers, mint (Life Savers Inc) (1)	7	30	2										
Life Savers, original assorted flavors (Life Savers Inc) (1)	9	40	2										
Milk chocolate (Hershey), 1oz (30g)	160	670	17		●		○				○		
Mr Goodbar (Hershey), 1½oz (40g)	210	880	18	○	●		○				○		○
Peanut-butter cups (Reese's), 2 pieces	190	800	18	○	●								○
Raisinets (Ward Johnson Inc), 1oz (30g)	100	420	14		●		○	○					
Real chocolate-covered mints (Brach's), 1oz (30g)	140	590	28		○								
Spearmint gum (Wrigley's), 1 piece	10	40	2										